I Used to Have Type I Diabetes

Kiss My Islets

by

Ellen Berty

First published by AuthorHouse 04/26/04

ISBN: 1-4184-2010-7 (e-book)
ISBN: 1-4184-2011-5 (Paperback)

Printed in the United States of America
Bloomington, IN

This book is printed on acid free paper.

TABLE OF CONTENTS

PREFACE

Having diabetes is like balancing on a high tightrope while carrying two huge, heavy, and unbalanced suitcases without a net below! And, throughout the balancing act, things get continually packed and unpacked from the suitcases.

After almost forty years and 22,000 shots of insulin, I can say that I no longer have Type 1 diabetes. As recently as five years ago, only those who received a pancreas transplant could say that. However, pancreas transplants are major surgery with all of the accompanying risks. On June 14, 2001, I had an islet cell transplant, an experimental procedure where the islets of Langerhans, which produce insulin, are taken from a donor pancreas and placed in the liver of a person with Type I diabetes.

This book is the story of my experience with diabetes including all the highs and lows, the islet cell procedure, and what a difference this has made in my life.

DEDICATION

I dedicate this book to my heroes; my husband, Peter, who has saved my life many times, and my doctor, Dave Harlan, who drastically improved it.

FOREWORD

I don't have diabetes. Though treating people with diabetes and finding ways to prevent or cure the disease have been my professional goals, I can never fully appreciate what it is like to live with the disease. Ellen Berty, with her inimitable combination of humor, energy, persistence, and real courage, describes life with diabetes and her experiences leading up to, during, and after her islet transplant received at the National Institutes of Health.

Ellen's stories will ring all-too-familiar to many people who have diabetes. In my own experience treating patients, I've heard many similar tales—sometimes funny but often disturbing or frightening. One that hit home happened when I was talking to a patient about the difficulties conducting an islet transplant study. The hard part, I said, was not knowing when we might get the call to isolate islets, which meant that my life could be disrupted at any time of day or night, any day of the week. The patient told me that is exactly what life with diabetes is all about! Having diabetes means never knowing when the disease will unpredictably disrupt life because blood sugar is too high or too low. Ellen recounts many such episodes. But she also explains the wonderful advances in the treatment of type 1 diabetes she's lived through—and most recently and dramatically, her islet transplant.

The islet transplant field has made great strides, led by indomitable researchers who persisted when experts said their efforts were hopeless. Many of these researchers are my heroes: Paul Lacy, David Scharp, Camillo Ricordi, Ray Rajotte, James Shapiro, and others. Comparing islet transplantation to powered flight, Drs. Lacy, Scharp, Ricordi, and their collaborators showed some years ago that islet transplantation held great promise and could work just as the Wright Brothers showed in 1903 that heavier-than-air powered flight could work. In 2000, the team led by Dr. James Shapiro at the University of Alberta in Edmonton, Canada, showed that islet transplantation was becoming more reliable, just as Charles Lindbergh ushered in the promise of air travel when he made the first solo flight across the Atlantic in 1927. Yet, flight did not become sufficiently safe and reliable to be a widely used mode of transportation until the mid-1930s, more than 30 years after the Wright Brothers "proof of concept" flight at Kitty Hawk.

Like powered flight, islet transplantation has now been shown to work with some reliability, when blood sugar control is used as the sole measure of success. As a physician, however, I believe that success should be defined more broadly. Ellen tells of complications such as high blood pressure, high cholesterol, infections, and other problems she has experienced in the few years after her islet transplant. These side effects are common in those who take the powerful cocktail of anti-rejection drugs that prevent the immune system from rejecting donated tissue.

There is much we still need to learn. We do not know how long the transplanted islets will survive or whether the transplant will be safe in the long-term (for example, can islets in the liver lead to liver damage down the road?). In addition, we do not know whether, on balance, we truly improve the lives of most people who undergo this procedure. Perhaps the most important unanswered question of all is: Does an islet transplant extend the life of the recipient? As we await answers, which will come only through further investigation, diabetes research can now focus on overcoming the hurdles that still limit islet transplantation: the inadequate number of organ donors, the still-too unpredictable islet isolation procedure, and the imperfect means currently available to prevent islet rejection (current anti-rejection medicines are not completely effective and are still, for many, simply too toxic).

By truly partnering with Ellen Berty and others who volunteer with full knowledge of the risks associated with medical research, we will overcome these remaining hurdles. For this and many other reasons, I believe Ellen as well as her husband Peter, her family, and her friends who have supported her through the years should be recognized as heroes in the war to conquer diabetes. This war is a team effort, and as a team, we will win that war. On that day, as Lewellys Barker told Sir Frederick Banting regarding the discovery of insulin in 1921, there will be "glory enough for all!"

David M. Harlan, M.D.
National Institutes of Health

Chapter 1
MY DIAGNOSIS AND EARLY TREATMENT

In 1961, at a rebellious thirteen years of age, flu-like symptoms plagued me for many months. Constantly feeling tired caused me to miss a major portion of the eighth grade. My parents knew this was unusual behavior, because my energy level was always high and it was sometimes difficult even to slow me down. I needed frequent rests to complete assignments sent home by my teacher. For me, this wasn't really an unpleasant time, since I got to hang around with my mother and eat and drink throughout the day. I am the oldest of six children, and there was always plenty of food around. We purchased apples by the bushel and my father baked thirty-two loaves of bread a week, always on Saturday morning. But no matter what or how much I ate, I didn't gain any weight. We were puzzled.

In addition to eating large quantities of food, I also was drinking lots of liquids and urinating frequently. My family would often go on outings, which, for a family of eight, was a masterful accomplishment. My mother had to make sure that all six of us had dressed properly, eaten recently, had a drink, and gone to the bathroom. And this was just to go grocery shopping! Despite her best-laid plans, as soon as we would arrive at the store I would immediately have to rush to the bathroom. My nine-year-old brother, Tom, saw humor in this ongoing situation and would tell my mother: "Ellen has to go again!"

In attempting to discover the root of the problem, my mother and I would visit the doctor's office every week. The office was only two blocks away, but this would tire me out tremendously. Every time, the doctor would inevitably say, "It's just a virus, and recovery will come in time." Then he would send us home to wait for my recovery. We would return after another week with no improvement and repeat the whole process, again and again. This continued from early September until March. My worst symptom was fatigue, and so rest was the treatment.

After six months of this routine, we finally changed doctors. My deteriorating vision prompted the change. A quick blood test at the new doctor's office confirmed his suspicion. My mother and I were sitting in the doctor's office anxiously waiting for the results when he entered the room and announced, "Young lady, you have diabetes."

My first thoughts were, "OK, what medicine is used to treat this disease, and how long will it last?" His next words were overwhelming: "This is a chronic disease you will have for the rest of your life." Up to this point in my short life, the doctor had always fixed everything right away. This was not the way it was supposed to be. My family shared my initial feelings of helplessness and sense of great ignorance. What exactly was this disease and how would we deal with it? What was the cause? Is it contagious? What do we have to do? Will my brothers and sisters get it, too? How about my parents? What is the treatment? What were the long-term implications? What was the cure? There is no cure? How long before a cure will be discovered? The doctor patiently explained that my pancreas

2

was not producing the insulin needed to process the sugars in food. Because my body was not using the sugars in food, it stayed in my blood and eventually spilled over into my urine. Since my body was not making insulin, I would have to put it there myself. I thought, "I can handle this—an insulin pill isn't too bad." But we left the doctor's office that day with many of our questions still unanswered.

After my diagnosis, I was immediately hospitalized and started insulin treatment. I experienced a rude awakening when the realization hit me that insulin was not taken in the form of a pill. It came in a shot. A shot I would have to give myself every single day for the rest of my life in order to live.

Through education and training, we learned a lot about diabetes, and some of our questions were answered. My parents told me later that they really felt they should have recognized my symptoms as signs of diabetes. Sure, they had heard about it, but only from a maternal great aunt who had Type 2 diabetes, a less severe form of diabetes where the body still produces some insulin but the ability to use it effectively is diminished or it is not enough. Oral medications were used to control her diabetes. The only treatment for Type I diabetes, insulin, had only been discovered forty years earlier. Before insulin, patients were literally starved to death in an effort to keep their blood sugars down and typically only lived for a short time after their islets stopped producing insulin. Eating normally after diagnosis usually resulted in a quicker death. So now when my doctors told me that my body didn't make insulin anymore, at least there was a treatment that would allow me to live. Because the body needs insulin to process the sugars in food, I would have to inject that insulin in order to survive. However, they couldn't tell me exactly what caused my body to stop making insulin. The medical professionals told us I would have to balance insulin, food, and exercise to achieve the proper level of sugar in my body. As for a cure, all they could tell me was this: "We think that one day there will be a cure, but there is not one available now. Researchers are trying to discover the cause and the cure, and we hope they will have the answers soon. We foresee this happening in the near future." When I tried to pin them down to a more specific timeline, they said that maybe a cure would be discovered within the next ten years. That seemed like a long time to me at thirteen. And of course, I didn't know that I would actually have to wait much longer.

This was a frightening disease for my parents. I was a teenager, so I just accepted it and moved on. My parents understood more about the long-term and life-threatening complications than I did. For me, long term meant next week. Recently my mother told me that at the time of my diagnosis, she desperately wished that it was she, not me that had diabetes. Although I didn't yet grasp the long-term implications, she understood what might lie ahead. If diabetes remains uncontrolled and blood sugars are high, this can cause many severe complications—including amputation, blindness, kidney failure, cardiac difficulties, and death. Many women with diabetes are unable to have children due to problems with conception, and difficulties maintaining proper blood sugar levels when they are pregnant. Even then, unless the blood sugar is very tightly controlled during pregnancy, there is a higher risk of fetal death or birth defects. Low blood sugars were another extreme that could result in unconsciousness and other complications, especially if the patient was not aware that her blood sugar was dropping. All of these dire possibilities were very real complications that my parents desperately hoped I would not have to face.

For me though, the situation still held some novelty. After a week in the hospital, the oranges I used when practicing my insulin shots became fully saturated. Those oranges certainly got a lot of insulin! When my brothers and sisters came to visit me in the hospital, I shared this new and exciting trick with them—big stuff for a thirteen-year-old. In the hospital, there were many sessions devoted to nutrition education, both for my parents and myself. The doctors explained an exchange system for food calculations. With this system, there were different categories of food, such as, fruits and vegetables, starches, and meats. Of course, in the hospital the only food available to me was already calculated and balanced with my insulin. Once I started taking insulin, and balancing my food, my health improved dramatically. My old energy returned, and I was up and ready to go again.

I returned to school and successfully completed eighth grade. The kids at school welcomed me back and asked how I was feeling. They really didn't know much about diabetes, and I was very reluctant to give them any details. Diabetes was a somewhat mysterious disease that did not affect many people at that time. The general public was generally not very knowledgeable about diabetes unless they were directly involved with someone who had the disease. For my friends in eighth grade, it was an unknown disease that they thought was scary and might possibly be something they could catch from me. I was not very confident in my knowledge of diabetes and was unwilling to share what little I did know with them. My quick response to their questions was "I'm fine," by which I clearly meant that I wanted that statement to end that topic of conversation. Certainly, they never knew about my daily injections and that I tested my urine for how much sugar was "spilling." That would make me different, and my desire was to be the same. At that point, I was prescribed NPH insulin (neutral protamine Hagedorn, an insulin suspension). This is a slow release type of insulin that works over an eight to twenty-four hour period. I only needed to take one shot each morning, so I didn't have to disclose my secret during the school day.

On more than one occasion, my secret almost got out. I regularly needed to collect my urine for a 24-hour period to check how my kidneys were functioning. During one of those collection periods, as I entered the house after a day in high school, my mother called out, "Ellen, have you gone to the bathroom yet?" She didn't realize that a prospective boyfriend had walked me home, carried my books, and was standing right next to me. I was mortified! There was no way I was willing to explain anything to this new recruit. I just shrugged my shoulders and gave him the look that all teenagers exchange when their parents say something uncomfortably parental.

There were changes in my home because of my diabetes. I had a little area in the kitchen where I kept all my supplies. "Ellen's cabinet" held my food, needles, glass syringes, and urine testing equipment. This cabinet was right next to the refrigerator, in which a small section of a shelf was reserved for my insulin. This was long before the days of disposable needles and syringes, the availability of various kinds of insulin, and home blood glucose (sugar) meters. Those major improvements were not available in 1961. Boiling my glass syringes to sterilize them and sharpening needles became part of my routine. Urine testing was the only self-monitoring system available. Of course, by the time sugar had spilled into my urine, my glucose level had already been high for quite a while. I would faithfully record the results and take the information to my medical appointments. A blood test was done at the doctor's office on each visit to determine the actual level of sugar in my blood at that time. Blood sugar levels are much more accurate than urine sugars but these were only available at the doctor's office. Adjustments to my insulin levels and food were made depending on those results and the data I shared.

My parents were very supportive during this learning period. Their support made the disease much easier to accept, and it become part of our daily lives. They always encouraged all of their children to be independent, and my situation was no exception, although it was slightly different. In my little corner of the kitchen, I had privacy from my siblings while taking my shot or recording my results. My parents always let me take care of everything, but were there to keep an eye on things and offer support when I needed it. They worked with me to figure out my food exchanges, but they never said, "You can't have that." They made sure healthy meals and snacks were available to the whole family. My mother always seemed to be busy in the kitchen when I was there giving myself a shot, and with a family of eight, it was not difficult for her to find something to do in the kitchen.

My parents educated themselves—and me—about diabetes. They joined the American Diabetes Association. Through membership in this organization, I received a monthly magazine with a special section geared toward children with diabetes. We would all read this magazine and discuss articles and information. My mother always took me to my doctor appointments, with various assortments of siblings forced to accompany us. One of the major things my family did for me was to give up desserts. Before my diagnosis, we always had meat, potatoes, vegetables, and a dessert for every dinner. After my diagnosis, dessert changed to canned fruit. A sugar-free gelatin, called "Dezerta," was my dessert. Cakes, pies, ice cream, and cookies disappeared from our home. My seven-year-old sister Paula thought this was unfair because I still got to have dessert. One taste of my Dezerta, however, and she quickly changed her mind.

During the six months I was treated for the "flu" instead of diabetes, I developed cataracts as a result of having very high blood sugars over such a long period of time. My ophthalmologist told me that cataracts are a film across the lens of the eye. My vision had slowly been deteriorating as the white film grew and clouded my vision. Surgery to remove the cataracts had to wait until the cataracts were "ripe." My vision continued to deteriorate until the ripening process was finished in 1964, when I was sixteen years old. The procedure used was called "needling," which involved pushing the cataracts to the viscera behind the eye. Viscera is a collective term used to describe the internal organs. This was a new procedure then. Previously, the treatment meant lying with sandbags on either side of your head for days after surgery. This was definitely an improvement since no sandbags were involved and I had a relatively short hospital stay. Doctors only worked on one eye at a time. The second cataract ripened by 1967, and the second operation was performed when I was nineteen years old. While in the hospital many people visited because it was almost unheard of for anyone so young to have cataract surgery. Most other patients were in their sixties or seventies.

After the first surgery, I had to wear extremely thick glasses that resembled the bottom of a glass Coca-Cola bottle. Back then, Coke bottles were made of glass, not plastic. I called them my "magic glasses" because they really magnified my eyes. And to me, they were magic, because the world was now visible to me. It looked like everything had been washed. Walking down the street, I read aloud all the street signs, store names, and billboards that had been missing from my sight for years. People glanced in my direction with quizzical looks on their faces as they passed me on the street.

About ten years after the "needling" operation, I had laser surgery to zap the cataracts off my lenses. This was a much easier procedure that was done on an outpatient basis. They simply "zapped" my eyes. This time, recovery was quick, and I left the facility shortly afterwards.

Contact lenses arrived on the scene for me shortly after that. Initially, ten minutes was all my eyes could stand of these new, hard lenses. I was slowly able to increase the time my eyes would tolerate the lenses. I spent many hours searching for contacts that had fallen out. The first time I lost a contact, it had rolled to the back of my finger, and I had inadvertently flung it across the room. Luckily, that extensive search ended fruitfully.

As contact options expanded, I decided to try extended-wear soft contacts that could be left in for days. My real motivation was my desire to see my dreams. During one night, when I woke up a little but was still dazed and sleepy, I felt something on the roof of my mouth. Thinking it was a piece of onion, I moved it down with my tongue and swallowed. Awaking in the morning, things on one side of the room definitely looked clearer than the other. Then I concluded that my contact was missing. Immediately realizing it was not an onion that had been in my mouth the night before, I decided not to look for that contact.

Another contact bit the dust and was never seen again when my thirteen-year old brother was standing with me in a phone booth. A college break had given me some time to visit with my family in Charleston, West Virginia. My brother, Phil, and I were out doing an errand, and squeezed into a phone booth to call home and ask a question. When I discovered my contact had fallen out I said, "Freeze. Don't move." My brother readily complied, thinking this was some sort of new college game. But the all too familiar search then began. After an extensive investigation of our clothing, the walls, and even the phone, we finally gave up. As we stepped out of the booth, we glanced down where Phil had been standing and saw the shattered pieces of my hard contact.

Sometimes I felt as if I was doing research for the contact lens manufactures on the extremes their products could tolerate. While traveling in the frigid regions of northern New York state, I had mistakenly left my soft contacts in the car overnight. I retrieved my frozen contacts in the morning and rushed inside to wait for the ice to melt. Luckily, my contacts eventually did thaw and were once again wearable.

Throughout my high school and college days I strove to keep my diabetes hidden from everyone. I wanted to be just like everyone else. So, in high school I was a cheerleader, I participated in student government and acting, and even hung out at the local pizza parlor. I could take my insulin shot at home before I went to school, so no one knew about that. Privacy in the bathroom stalls afforded me the opportunity to check my urine undetected by anyone else. Not experiencing any low blood sugars, I successfully kept my diabetes hidden. The school nurse knew about my disease, but her usual treatment of any illness I experienced at school was to send me home. My attendance was good and I rarely missed school. I enjoyed high school and loved all the social activities involved with my friends. I took my lunch to school so I could be in control of the food I ate. Embarrassment caused me to conduct all my medical activities behind closed doors.

Despite all my efforts, one of those doors was opened while I was attending college in 1970 and living in a house with three other women. One housemate,

Becky, walked into the bathroom while I was injecting the needle into my arm. Her eyes widened in amazement, and she backed out of the room and closed the door. My response—or rather lack of it—was complete silence. Becky never spoke about the incident to me. I was certain that my housemates thought that I was using drugs and, of course, that was true. However, my drug was not illegal, as they probably presumed. This discovery still did not cause me to reveal my secret. I wanted to keep my diabetes private and handle everything myself. Telling people about my disease would invade my privacy and I did not want sympathy. I felt confident that I did not need anyone's help.

While in graduate school, my friend and housemate Kim came to visit me after a diabetes-related incident resulted in hospitalization. She did not know I had diabetes and was very surprised to learn the reason for my stay in the hospital. After her visit, I felt a little more willing to discuss diabetes with her. She had a base of knowledge about diabetes because her father was a doctor and she immediately called him before I was released from the hospital. That was essentially my "coming out" party.

At about this time, Peter Berty came into my life. During an unusually warm spell over the Christmas holidays, we met at a picnic at a mutual friend's farm. We realized we were both attending the same university and decided to get together once we returned to school. I was a graduate student in education and he was an undergraduate studying psychology. Our first date was a portent of things to come. He was able to get front row tickets to "Jesus Christ Superstar." The previous night I had neglected to remove my contacts before falling asleep. The next morning, my eyes had swollen shut. Calling Pete, I begged him to drive me to the hospital. That was just the first of many times he has come to my rescue. The doctors were able to remove the contacts, but it was extremely painful to open my eyes. I stayed in bed that evening and missed our first date.

Pete and I had been dating for almost eleven months when we started discussing marriage. As soon as we began that discussion, I told him there was something he needed to know. I'm sure he felt some apprehension as he waited for what was to come. The announcement that I had diabetes came as a surprise. He didn't know much about the disease and had never known anyone else with diabetes. He had noticed that I didn't eat desserts and that I maintained a healthy diet. He wondered how this might affect our life together, but we were in love and didn't view the issue as a major hurdle to our marriage. At that point, he certainly didn't realize that 25 years later he would have to get up at 4 a.m. to give me a shot that would save my life. I was doing well with the disease at this point, so diabetes really was no big deal to him or to me.

Chapter 2
TRAVELING WITH DIABETES

Throughout my forty years with diabetes I never let it stop me from doing anything. It certainly did cause me to have to make many accommodations and adjustments, but it never prevented me from engaging in any activity or going anywhere. One of the things that required lots of adjustments, special accommodations, and precautions was travel. My husband and I have traveled in the United States, Canada, Europe, and South America. Adventures in these places have caused to me to learn some valuable lessons.

Precautions

Before traveling anywhere, I always carried prescriptions for insulin, needles, and syringes as well as test strips and an extra meter with spare batteries. I also carried a letter from my doctor explaining that I had diabetes. Wearing a medic-alert bracelet also is a necessary precaution that can be a life saver. Identification (passport/driver's license) is an important thing to have on your person. When traveling to a foreign country, I always tried to carry a translation of my doctor's letter. With the help of the Internet, it is now possible to have text translated online. Although the result does not always reflect the particular vernacular and idiosyncrasy of the language, at least the general idea can be translated. Even carrying a simple list of critical terms such as diabetes, insulin, syringe, needles, illness, doctor, etc. may be helpful.

Extra backup supplies are an important part of traveling. Packing twice as much as what will actually be needed is a good idea. Keeping supplies in two separate places is essential. One set of supplies should be kept on your person or in your carry-on luggage, if flying. Carrying supplies in zippered pockets can prevent lost bottles of insulin while hiking, skiing, boating, biking, or even just sitting. Candy and glucose tablets also were an essential part of my travel kit.

Traveler's insurance can be a lifesaver in an emergency. Not only can they arrange for special transport out of a location where adequate emergency assistance may not be available, but they also can try to locate medication if your supply is lost or stolen.

Searches

When my needles and syringes were discovered by border patrols or airport security this always piqued their curiosity and resulted in a much more extensive search of both my belongings and myself. They were suspicious of possible drug use and distribution. After finishing graduate school in 1972, I traveled to Europe with a friend. Kim and I were off on an adventure with no set plans and limited financial resources. We frequently hitchhiked to get from one place to another. We decided to go to Amsterdam and posted a sign at the youth hostel in Wiesbaden, Germany asking for a ride. A few days later we got an offer that we accepted. All of our belongings were in backpacks that we threw into the trunk of a car owned by a couple who were traveling around Europe. We were joined by a young German who also wished to go to Amsterdam. We were stopped at the border crossing into Holland. As the border patrol looked into the car, they asked us all to get out and they began a search. They emptied my backpack and were very excited to find my needles and syringes. They were obviously searching for drugs. I produced a letter from my doctor, explaining my condition and the necessity for needles and syringes. Using many gestures, I attempted to demonstrate that I took insulin, not some illegal drug. This did not appear to satisfy them and they continued an extensive search of the whole car. They removed the back seat, took the hubcaps off the wheels, and looked into the gas tank and every other conceivable place that could possibly conceal drugs. We were each questioned extensively in their limited English and our extremely limited Dutch. Eventually after many, many hours and an unproductive search on their part, they allowed us to pass. We all breathed a sigh of relief and continued our journey.

Starting in December of 1976, my husband and I traveled extensively in South America for three months. After our adventures, we flew from Lima, Peru to Bogotá, Columbia. We planned our departure from Bogotá, Columbia back to the United States. We arrived at the airport looking very scruffy. We had worn the same few items of clothing for three months and they were now baggy because we had lost weight during our travels. No haircuts and travel-worn backpacks added to our scruffiness. We arrived on a flight from Lima along with a group of newly retired, wealthy people. We were 27 and 28. To say we looked a little different from the rest of the group was definitely an understatement. We were immediately taken out of the line of arriving passengers for a search when we arrived at the airport, as we looked very suspicious and likely to be transporting drugs. We were each taken into separate rooms; a female inspector accompanied me, and a male accompanied my husband. They went through everything in our packs and of course found my syringes. They asked many questions which I attempted to answer in my limited Spanish. Possibly due to the syringes or just because we fit their profile of drug smugglers; a full body search was conducted to assure that I was not concealing any illegal drugs in any of my body cavities. This was the first and only time I have experienced such a through examination by someone other than a medical professional. After completing the search, we were allowed to enter Columbia along with our unlikely travel companions.

Europe

While traveling in Spain with my college roommate my finger became infected after swimming in water close to where the septic system emptied into the sea. The infection was serious and required medical attention. My friend, Kim, spoke Spanish and was very helpful in finding out that we needed to go to the local hospital in order to see a doctor. We navigated our way around Barcelona and finally ended up at the hospital. Kim answered all the questions the receptionist at the hospital asked while I simply showed my finger whenever she nudged me. A few nurses and then some doctors looked at my finger. Finally, they put me in a wheelchair and pushed me into an operating room. They did not allow Kim, my translator and lifeline, to accompany me. I was on my own. This was very frightening because it was unknown what they were going to do to me. The possibility of amputation did cross my mind. Watching carefully as they examined the finger under some type of scope, I saw them produce all their instruments to do the surgery. Once I saw the surgical instruments, I was even more frightened as the amputation possibility loomed even closer. They were, of course, talking to me and each other, in Spanish, none of which I understood. They started to scrape the outer skin of my finger away. Since they had not started with a quick chop,

I was reassured and hopeful that maybe they were not going to amputate. They continued to scrape until they had removed all of the infected area. Whew! My finger would remain a part of my hand. "Gracias, gracias, gracias," was all I could say. They wrapped my finger with a gauze pad and then swaddled it in a huge white bandage and instructed me to keep the hand elevated. We received quite a few curious looks on the bus as I stood there with my middle finger elevated and wrapped in a gigantic white bandage.

RAGBRAI

Shortly after Pete and I were married, we lived in Des Moines, Iowa where he was earning his graduate degree at Drake University. The local newspaper, The Des Moines Register, sponsors a bike ride across Iowa every summer. It is known as the RAGBRAI (Register's Annual Great Bike Ride Across Iowa). This is a weeklong event that attracts thousands of riders every year. It has grown to such an extent that they now use a lottery to limit the number of riders. In 1975, a group of us from my office decided that we could ride 450 miles in 7 days with 3,000 other bikers. The bicyclists often outnumbered the residents of the towns we biked through. People in these small towns considered it quite an honor (and an economic boost) to have the ride pass through their towns and happily and graciously supplied dinners for all the bikers for a nominal fee. The newspaper carried all the gear in big semi trucks and we camped in the parks. One morning, while in the bathroom taking my shot, I dropped my bottle of insulin. The crash on the tile floor shattered my bottle into a least a hundred pieces. My spare bottle was in the truck that had already left for that day's final destination. Realizing there was no way I could continue without my insulin, I hesitantly approached a townsperson who had been working on breakfast. After explaining the situation, he immediately offered to drive me to the nearest town that had a drug store. Once

17

at the store, I begged the pharmacist for more insulin. Not having a prescription, he was somewhat reluctant to supply the insulin. Once I shared all the details, he did agree. The townsperson drove me back to my bike at the park and I was once again on my way.

The wrist story

My husband Pete and I had flown to Hungary to join a ski club on their annual ski trip in January of 2000. From Veszprem, we traveled 8 hours by bus to the Dolomites in Italy with a group of 100 skiers. They welcomed us warmly into their group and we enjoyed many hours of fun with them. We skied the slopes surrounding the village of Sappada where majestic views greeted us in every direction. Above the ski slopes, bare rocks piled to the 7,000-foot summits surrounding the valley. On the afternoon of our fifth and last day, I decided to go ice-skating. I had a wonderful time skating to Italian rock music at an outdoor rink. At times, I was the only one on the whole rink. All in all, this was a peaceful and pleasant scene. However, the shadow of doom lingered nearby. This is my story; a story of surprise, ache, suspense, and perseverance.

At around 4:30, the skiers returned to the bus to go back to our hotel. As they passed the rink, they stopped to talk with me. Pete came by and I skated over to talk with him. While standing there talking, I didn't notice that there was a little, sloping lip on the edge of the ice. My skates went over the lip, I lost my balance and fell straight down. I tried to cushion the fall with my hands. I ended up sitting on the edge of the ice while pain shot through my wrist. Pete asked what he could do to help. I slowly stated that my wrist was broken. Knowing me well after 27 years of marriage, he said that I should not exaggerate and maybe it wasn't that bad, but I convinced him. I stayed seated on the ice as he went to get my boots

18

from the bus. On the way, he told the rink manager (using pantomime) that I had broken a bone and needed an ambulance (ambulanza).

In the meantime, Olga (a doctor who was with our skiing group) came over to offer her assistance. She removed my mitten and looked at my grotesquely misshapen and swollen wrist and hand. She immediately emitted a loud moan. This really was not very encouraging! She tried to remove my rings. My fingers were already swollen but with some cream that someone provided, she manipulated my rings until they come off. She also removed my medical alert bracelet from around my swollen wrist. The skating rink attendant came over, looked at my wrist and said "ambulanza." The ambulance had to be called from Auronzo (the nearest town with a hospital), which was 18 miles away. It arrived at about 5:30. While waiting, several returning skiers offered me pálinka (Hungarian plum brandy). That stuff burned enough to make me forget about my wrist momentarily.

The ambulance took Pete and me over winding mountain roads through small towns where, at some points, only one car could fit between the buildings (or so I am told). We arrived at the hospital at about 6 p.m. They took x-rays and said "broken." They informed us that their hospital was only for infectious diseases. We must go to Cortina d'Ampezzo where there was an orthopedic hospital. Cortina was 22 miles further but the same ambulance could not take us there. They had to send their own ambulance.

An hour after we arrived in Auronzo, an ambulance pulled in from Cortina. Again we traveled on mountainous, winding roads. Finally, after a 40-minute ride, we arrived at the orthopedic hospital in Cortina. Now the ambulance drivers wanted to be paid. The first ambulance took our insurance card (which was a pleasant surprise). We did not have enough lira—we planned to leave the country the next morning. Pete was able to communicate that he could get money at a bank machine (bancomat). They took him in the ambulance to the bancomat where he got the lira and paid the driver. He asked to be taken back to the hospital. They informed him that they could not do that since it was no longer an emergency! Pete tried to get a taxi but none were available possibly because of the crowds in town for the World Cup skiing competition. So he started to walk back in the direction of the hospital, not exactly sure of the route. Also, now he was carrying a bundle of extra ski clothes because we had not had a chance to change. He finally made it back to the hospital in about half an hour after only one wrong turn!

Meanwhile, back at the hospital (at about 7:45 p.m.), I attempted to communicate using my five words of Italian. Any combination of "good day", "goodbye", "yes", "good", and "thanks" still left only limited possibilities. It is a very good thing that I am usually a winner in Charades! They took me right into the emergency room and treated me immediately. They had to take new x-rays as we left the earlier ones at the first hospital. They said, "broken" and began their work.

First, they removed all my remaining layers of ski clothes. Five layers later, they were ready to start. I got a local anesthetic injected directly into the back of my swollen hand (and that smarts). It took teamwork to set the bone. Two nurses pulled in opposite directions on my hand and arm, while the doctor put his weight on my bone and pushed it back into place. He put on a plaster cast and sent me back for yet another x-ray to make sure it was set correctly. Once it was set the pain was considerably less. The x-ray was "perfetto" and he put on the rest of the cast above my elbow, halfway to my shoulder. The doctor tried to communicate to me that I must spend the night. I knew that our chartered bus would depart from Italy for Hungary at 9 the next morning. We were 40 miles west of our hotel and the bus would be heading east.

He said I should take another bus. I told him there was no other bus. He said I must stay. I said I can not. He said I should take a plane. I just did not seem to be getting my message across! By a series of pantomimes, he was able to let me know that it was dangerous for me to travel as the bone setting was fragile and he was worried about swelling. Well, he convinced me!

They took me up to a room and tried to find a doctor who spoke English. They were somewhat successful. I tried to inform them about the medications I took. Throughout this entire interaction the doctor left frequently when she was apparently stumped by some word. I was not sure where she went or whether she talked with someone or simply looked in the dictionary but she usually returned with another question. I, of course, had no medication with me as everything was back in the hotel 40 miles away! I took medication for a thyroid condition. They flat out said they just did not have that. I take that medication in the morning so I could wait until Pete could bring this to me in the morning. We tried to establish what my diabetes needs were. I tried to explain about Lente insulin (fast acting). I quickly gave up on this and tried for a simple NPH routine (slow acting). They had this type of insulin and I wrote the amount down. Now, at last, my blood sugars would be more manageable and the danger of hyperglycemia would be abated. They did take frequent blood sugars. I also have glaucoma and require eye drops to decrease pressure in my eyes. They did not have the same specific kind but they had a substitute medication. They gave me this and told me to let them know if it caused pain.

Pete returned from paying the ambulance drivers and found me at about 8:30 p.m. I gave him all the details of the events he had missed. He decided I was settled in and he would return, somehow, someway in the morning. The doctor told him that I would be x-rayed again in the morning and I would be allowed to leave by 9:00 a.m.—if it looked good. Otherwise, I'd have to stay!

He then went off to look for food and called Anikó and Zoli (a couple in our group who had a cell phone) to let them know what was happening. At about 9:30 p.m., he took a $125 taxi ride back to our hotel and tried to make arrangements for the next morning.

Meanwhile, at the hospital, I had finally settled in and tried to sleep. I removed my contacts and placed them in drinking cups. My glasses were back at the hotel. So now, not only can I not understand what people are saying, I can no longer see them! My roommate, who spoke no English, got ready for bed and then came over to me and said something and pounded on the table with the palm of her hand. I finally figured out that she was telling me that if I had any trouble during the night, I should just pound on the table and she would help me. How sweet!

Shortly after that, my hand felt very cold and I had pain in my wrist (no surprise) but also at my elbow. I let the nurse know this by placing her hand on top of mine. She called a few more people who come in, felt my hand, and carried on an animated discussion. They left and called the doctor. She also came and felt my hand. Then a nurse came in with a wheelchair. She indicated I should get in the chair. I asked her why and she said "emergenze." What am I to do? I got in the chair and went along for the ride.

Back in the emergency room, they turned my head away from what they were doing. I heard the saw as they cut open the cast and pried it apart to accommodate the swelling. I was sitting in the chair and I said, "I feel like I am going to faint." The doctor and another semi-English speaker looked at each other and tried to figure out the word "feel." They raised their eyebrows and shrugged their shoulders. That's when I fainted. (The only other time I fainted was when I watched a cast being removed from my son's leg. Must be something about that saw.) I came to on a stretcher and I think they said something that sounded somewhat like my name. They thought I had suffered a heart attack, and took an EKG. There was another animated discussion afterward and they repeatedly asked "medicina pressure?" I eventually figured out that they were asking if I took blood pressure medicine. I said "no" and then they did another EKG. The results of this one were good and I was wheeled back to my room.

Yeah! Rest at last! I went to the bathroom, which is down the hall. The nurse escorted me but left me there. Of course, I couldn't see and while I attempted to locate my room, the nurse found me wandering toward another room. She steered me in the right direction. I could not sleep and tried to get something for pain. After many gestures and trips in and out of the room, the nurse finally returned with a shot. I think that they had to call the doctor to get permission to give the shot even though the doctor had, I thought, communicated to me that I could have one if needed.

Meanwhile, Pete arrived back at the hotel at around 11:00 p.m. (having had only a chocolate bar for dinner and it was white chocolate, not even real chocolate!) and found that the ski group's goodbye party was winding down. János, the "ski camp" director, took him to Olga's room (she and her family had come by car).

23

She agreed with his proposal for the following morning, which was that, after breakfast, her children (ages 11 and 13) would ride on the bus in our place while she and her husband took Pete to pick me up. Next, they went to Jutka's room to get some sandwiches she made for Pete. (Jutka is the only person we knew before the trip.) Finally, Pete was back in our room where he was starving, his eyes hurt from dried out contacts, and he was overheated in his ski clothes. He was faced with a dilemma—which pain to relieve first. Those who know him won't be surprised that, first, he ate. After three he packed up our things, which were scattered all over the room, he managed to get 3 hours of sleep.

At the hospital, finally, it was morning. They took me back down to x-ray for another picture. Things looked good and they put on another layer of cast to cover where they had to open it during the night. Pete and Olga were in my room when I returned at about 9:30 a.m. (Olga's husband, Karcsi, was waiting in the car.) It took another hour and a half to get a copy of the x-rays and the doctor's report, but we finally left to meet the bus! Cell phones afforded us the luxury of speaking with those on the bus. The bus had a scheduled two-hour stop in Tarvisio (near the Austrian border) for shopping. They graciously waited an additional hour for us to catch them.

The accident happened on Friday afternoon. We were scheduled to leave Hungary on the following Tuesday (January 25). We boarded the plane with no further incident. However, almost four hours into the flight, when we were over the Atlantic, there was an announcement, in Hungarian, from the pilot stating something about Budapest. I, with some hesitation, asked Pete what it was about. He said that the New York airport was closed due to a major snowstorm and that we were turning around and going back to Budapest!! By now, my hand had swollen out of the cast due to the low pressure in the cabin. We ended up back in Budapest. We had traveled almost eight hours in the plane and we had returned to where we started! We spent the night in a hotel and the next day started as a repeat of the previous day—same airport, same flight, same food, same movies, same swelling, but this time we actually arrived in New York after a 9 hour flight. Our connecting flight was cancelled but a later one was delayed only for a few hours. Eventually, we did arrive back in Arlington, Virginia after we had been awake for 24 hours.

After being a squeaky wheel with my HMO, I managed to get an appointment with an orthopedic doctor early the next day. Here it was different since we at least spoke the same language. After more x-rays the doctor recommended that the broken bones be pinned together and that an external apparatus (that would be screwed into the bones of my hand and arm) replace the cast. Surgery went well and afterwards I had more flexibility in my fingers and elbow. Scars remain on my arm and wrist but I now have almost full range of motion in my wrist.

Diabetes was an essential part of the entire treatment plan throughout this experience with my wrist. Stress and trauma definitely had an impact on my blood sugars. It was necessary to monitor my blood sugars more frequently and to adjust my insulin levels accordingly. And of course, added to that, were all the new and unusual foods that had to be calculated. Even in Italy, where it was much more difficult for me to manage, considering the language barrier, it was possible.

South America

While in South America, my husband, Pete, my brother, Tom, and I traveled by bus to Medellin, Columbia. We had befriended a local woman on the bus who was moving to Medellin and had all of her belongings with her. She had many high quality suitcases and appeared to be wealthy, at least by local standards. As we exited the bus, she flagged down a taxi and put everything into the trunk except for a small bag that she held. She walked over to us to invite us to stay at the same hotel where she was going, but the place sounded too expensive for our budget. She said goodbye, wished us well, and returned to where her taxi had been. Unfortunately, her taxi had quietly departed without her but with all of her belongings. She was very upset and cried that she must get to the police station. She begged us to guard her remaining possession. We placed her small bag on top of our packs, and stood against a blank wall on the sidewalk across from the bus station with Pete and me on either side of the packs. Tom had accompanied the woman to the police station to function as a witness and for moral support. We were watching our packs very carefully as we had been warned about the many clever thieves in Medellin and we had just witnessed one of their thefts. We were certainly on "alert."

A man and a boy coming from opposite directions on the sidewalk bumped into each other right in front of us. Coins cascaded all over the sidewalk. When we stepped forward to observe what was happening, someone lifted the women's bag! We had only been distracted for a second. There were many people in front of the bus station, but none of them gave any warning or even an indication that they had seen either of these two thefts. We wondered if they might have been thugs in training. With great trepidation, we waited for Tom and the women to return from the police station. After telling her that we were unable to guard her only remaining suitcase, she was distraught. We left her in the care of the local police and quickly made plans to leave town. I was very grateful to be leaving with all my medical supplies still in my possession.

Another adventure in South America involved white water rafting on the Urubamba River, a tributary of the Amazon, in Peru. Pete's brother, Lászlo, was starting a rafting business and wanted to gain some experience with people who would be similar to potential customers, that is, people who were not skilled white-water rafters. Pete, my brother Tom, and I volunteered to be his crew on his maiden voyage with novices. We started above the tree line in southern Peru, portaged around an impassable section near Machu Picchu, then entered the "eyebrow of the jungle," the wettest part. Macaws were often spotted along the shore. Lush rain forests lined the banks of the winding river. The rushing waters, blue skies, and bright sun were material for an enticing travel poster. The scenery was breathtakingly beautiful. There were very few towns or settlements along the river due to the sometimes very steep slopes and sheer cliffs that dropped dramatically down to the river. There were a few places where it was possible to access the river and locals would be ashore. We were quite a sight floating on a raft, in our colorful life jackets and helmets. What a contrast to the locals who dressed only in earth tones. The natives would line up along the shore and shout "peligroso" and "muy peligroso." We, being complete novices, thought this was just a greeting and would wave back with a big smile on our faces. Lászlo eventually informed us that this really was a warning from the locals, and the word "peligroso" meant danger. We did encounter some danger as the river began to rise each night. It was the rainy season, and the rain that fell upstream from us accumulated and swelled the river. Several nights we had to break camp and move our tents back, farther away from the river, which was quickly encroaching on our campsite.

All of our belongings were in large waterproof bags that were tied securely to the raft. I had put my medical supplies into two separate bags. There were many rapids along the river and some were quite large. Rapids are rated according to their class. Class I-III are easy and fun, Class III-IV are considered exciting and require some skill to run. Class V-V+ are intense and heavy duty; skill is required to get through these rapids. Class VI is considered to be unrunable. Many of the rapids on this part of the Urubamba were Class V. We would stop upstream of the rapids and scout to see exactly which was the safest path. One set of rapids looked quite impressive from our scouting position. It was impossible to portage around the rapids (because of the thick forest that came right down to the banks) so we prepared to go ahead. We checked all the lines to make sure that the bags were tied tightly. We tried to avoid the rapids but the strong current of the river pulled us directly into them. We quickly went through the rapids and were overturned. The extremely strong force of the wave flipped the raft and threw all of us into the madly rushing river. The force tore off one of my shoes. Holding tightly to one of the ropes, I was able to maintain contact as the boat rushed through the rapids upside down dragging me behind it. My brother was caught under the boat and was struggling to reach the surface. Eventually, he was able to pull himself around underneath the boat by inching his way along the ropes and finally gasping up to the surface. Pete and László bailed from the boat when it was on its upward flip, and they caught up with us again in calmer waters. After regrouping, we assessed the damages. Amazingly, no one was injured. One bag had been torn from its mooring on the boat and was lost. We quickly looked in the remaining bags to determine exactly what was in the missing bag. I sighed with relief as we opened the bags with my medical supplies. Only one essential item was missing. The all important diarrhea medicine was gone. For Pete and I, who had been suffering from this malady, this was devastating news. That night we discussed how long it would be before we could obtain more medicine. We were a long way from any civilization downriver, and without the medicine our chance of becoming dehydrated increased dramatically. Pete and I decided to abandon the river trip at this point. We hiked back to the nearest hacienda where we were able to hitch a ride on a truck back to civilization. Tom and László opted to continue and traveled down to the Amazon for another 15 days on the raft.

While waiting for the bus to leave a small town in Peru, I decided to go for a walk because the upcoming trip would be long. Leaving all of my things with my husband and brother at the bus station, I started off with my candy and passport. We had asked numerous times what time the bus left. If we responded with something that indicated we thought that was too soon, the locals would then quickly adjust the time to later. If, instead, we indicated that the time was too late, they would respond with an earlier time. In reality, the bus left when it was full. It took us quite a while to figure this out and we missed a few buses in that learning process. This particular experience in Peru occurred before we had come to this realization. After wandering aimlessly around the curving streets of the town admiring the buildings and checking out the local people, I started heading in the direction that, I thought, was toward the bus. The realization that I was lost hit me only after recognizing that I was on the same street for a second time in a short period of time. I began to panic that I would miss the bus and it would leave without me, and Pete and Tom would be gone. My insulin would also be gone. My speed increased in proportion to my panic. Running, I asked people on the street "Bus?" with a quizzical look on my face and shrugged my shoulders. Not wanting to waste any time stopping, I never got any answers that I could understand. Finally, a woman pointed in the direction from which I had just come. I quickly turned and headed that way. Luckily the bus loomed ahead of me with only my husband and brother standing in front of the bus, keeping it from leaving, while waving and shouting at me to hurry up. Stumbling up the stairs, I collapsed in a seat, grateful to once again be united with both my family and supplies! The bus was full, and the driver had been trying to leave for several minutes.

We traveled to Machu Picchu in Peru to view the ancient Inca fortress city atop a high saddle between two peaks. It appears to have been home to about 1,000 people, perhaps the Inca elite, who may have lived there during part of the year to conduct religious ceremonies. The city features several temples that align with the sun at certain times of the year, demonstrating the Incas' remarkable grasp of astronomy—not to mention their construction skills. Stone walls on the finer buildings were laid without mortar; blocks of granite weighing several tons are fitted so precisely that a piece of paper will hardly fit into the joints. The city was mysteriously abandoned around the time of the Spanish conquest, in the 1500s. It was rediscovered in 1911 by American explorer Hiram Bingham, whose articles and photographs about it captivated millions. A road to the site was built in 1948, and reconstruction of the site opened the way for tourists.

The train from Cuzco to Aguas Calientes, which is near Machu Picchu, was always crowded with locals and with tourists who were ready to either hike up the mountain or travel to the top by bus. On the return trip to Cuzco, we were watching our luggage very carefully because this train was frequently targeted by very competent thieves. As we pulled into the station, a local couple sat facing a tourist couple across the aisle from us. The local man stood up, yanked a backpack from the overhead rack, and let it fall onto the tourist woman. As she reached up to protect herself, the local woman slit her purse and removed her wallet, while the local man apologized for dropping the backpack. The local couple immediately went to the door, and having timed it perfectly, got off just as the train stopped. All this happened very quickly, and of course, neither we nor the tourist couple had noticed what the local woman had accomplished during the commotion. However, by the time the crime was discovered, the thieves were lost in the crowd.

During all this distraction, someone reached in from the window of the train, or possibly through the air vent in the roof, and lifted a small piece of our luggage. We had been carefully watching all our luggage but briefly glanced away as we gathered our things to depart. In the bag that was stolen was a camera and my husband's diary from our travels, but not my medical supplies. Even our most diligent efforts were unsuccessful in stopping theft.

Reflecting on these adventures, I am reminded of my brother-in-law's words as he was attempting to arrange for a ride aboard a Peruvian Air Force helicopter so he could scout an inaccessible area to assess its whitewater rafting potential. Not surprisingly, the colonel in charge refused the request the first several times, but he finally agreed when Lászlo exclaimed with great emotion, "Without adventure, what is life?"

Chapter 3
LOWS

My life with diabetes gradually changed as the disease became more difficult to manage. For many years, I had experienced fairly good control with no complications and only occasional episodes of severe low blood sugar (called "hypoglycemia"). During 40 years of dealing with diabetes, I have experienced many hypoglycemic reactions. A hypoglycemic reaction happens when the level of glucose (sugar) in the blood drops to abnormally low levels. My glucose levels ranged as low as zero (or at least that was the number my blood sugar meter displayed). The average blood sugar for a person without diabetes is 100. In general, glucose is the fuel that provides energy for the cells to operate. Insulin is the hormone used to convert that fuel into energy. It is necessary to balance the amount of insulin and food, keeping in mind that a myriad of other things affect the balance. When there is too much insulin, hypoglycemia results and when there is not enough insulin, high blood sugar (or "hyperglycemia") is the result. The most obvious factors that lower my blood sugar, sometimes to dangerous levels, are the amount and kinds of food I eat, illness, and exercise. Other factors such as stress, both good and bad, weather conditions, and menstrual cycles also are part of the complex mix that are not always as obvious.

Exercise typically had a delayed affect on my blood sugars. A few hours after exercising my blood sugars would drop and I had to eat something to keep it up. This occurred even after adjusting for the exercise by decreasing my insulin intake. It took me quite a while to understand the delayed effect of exercise. After bike riding for forty to fifty miles, eating frequently, and monitoring my blood sugars levels, I would finish the ride in the late afternoon and measure my blood sugar. At this point, it was usually within the accepted range of low 100s even after eating much more than normal. I would eat dinner and take my blood sugar again before going to bed. Then, at three or four in the morning, I would awake in the midst of a hypoglycemic episode and find the bedclothes saturated with sweat (a typical side effect of hypoglycemia). Sometimes the reaction would not occur until the middle of the next day.

Surprisingly, air temperature and weather conditions also influenced my blood sugars. It took some detective work to discover that. One early spring night, I left the window next to the bed open a little bit. A nice, warm, gentle breeze was blowing when I went to bed. By the time my husband came to bed a few hours later, I was experiencing a severe hypoglycemic reaction. I was unconscious, sweating profusely, and just starting to have seizures. Pete had to give me a shot of glucagon to bring me around. Glucagon is a hormone produced by the alpha cells in the pancreas. It raises blood glucose very quickly. An injectable form of glucagon, available by prescription, is used to treat severe hypoglycemia. Raising my blood sugar immediately to bring me back to consciousness was the goal. When I started to come back around after one of those really severe reactions, it felt as if I was underwater and struggling to get to the surface. My brain would start to recover, and I could formulate in my mind what I wanted to say but I just couldn't get it out. (Apparently, the glucose was getting to my brain cells before it was getting to my muscles.) As my blood sugar started to rise I could finally start to form words, but I would still struggle to speak, and my speech would be unintelligible. This would slowly improve until I would eventually regain full consciousness and speech capability. At this point, the bedclothes would be completely drenched, as would my pajamas and the bed. So, the clothes had to be washed, the mattress dried out, and we had to sleep in another bed. All of that happened because the weather had changed and the air had gotten a little cooler. My body had to work a little harder to stay warm, and therefore used up more sugar. I ended up in dire circumstances even though my blood sugar was within the acceptable range before I went to bed.

Stress is another factor that affected my blood sugars. At one point, there was a lot of stress in my office because of an unbearable work situation. This caused lots of havoc on my blood sugars. I had to take a leave of absence from work until the situation improved. Good stress and excitement also have resulted in low blood sugars for me. These situations typically occurred in social situations with families and friends. Holiday gatherings, when meals aren't always ready on a regular schedule, have caused many a drop in blood sugar levels.

Unfortunately, time is a factor that I'm not always able to control. To provide just one example, we were on our way to a large dinner party at a friend's home. While traveling the congested Capital Beltway around Washington, D.C., to get to their home, we got stopped in a major traffic jam. Because we were going to dinner, I hadn't brought a lot of food with me. A couple pieces of candy weren't enough to keep my blood sugar up as we inched along in traffic. By the time we actually arrived at the house, I couldn't even get out of the car. My husband ran into the house to get some food, returned, and fed it to me. Eventually regaining enough coordination to move, I went into the house. Of course, everyone else had arrived long before and had waited for us before they sat down to dinner. It was one of many grand entrances that was very uncomfortable and embarrassing.

Food, of course, is another major cause of variations in blood sugar levels. It was often difficult for me to determine what had caused an especially elevated blood sugar level. Through experience, I discovered that many commercially-prepared foods and canned foods contain added sugars, including soups, tomato sauce, and other tomato-based foods. I learned to check all the ingredients on a package very carefully. Eating out in restaurants was a totally different ball game, however. My family members have never been fast food fans, so we easily avoided that kind of food. Taking a taste of a meal in a Lebanese restaurant on one occasion, I determined right away that a fair amount of sugar had been added to the dish. Asking at a restaurant if sugar is an ingredient in a dish could help avoid later unexpected elevated blood sugars.

Illness is another factor that caused wild swings in my blood sugar levels. On January 7, 1996 we were in the throes of a major blizzard. It was my husband's birthday, and I had not felt well all day. The flu was doing its thing with me. I had taken my regular amount of insulin, and even though I had not eaten very much during the day, my blood sugars were still running somewhat high. I went to bed around 7:00 p.m. because I was exhausted. After I had been in bed for a few hours, Pete heard some loud banging and came upstairs to investigate. I was in a coma, having seizures and covered with sweat. The banging he had heard was caused by my arms and legs hitting against the wall as I was flailing around during the seizures. He tried to wake me but this was impossible. He knew I was beyond candy so he gave a shot of glucagon. This was his first experience with glucagon and he was uncertain of how long the response time would be. After a couple of minutes, I was still not conscious so he called 911. The emergency people drove down snow covered roads to reach our home, and plowed through the snow to our door. Their snow covered clothing and boots left many puddles inside. By this time I was starting to come around and regained consciousness. The emergency personnel advised me to seek medical attention and have things checked out. They took me to the hospital where I stayed for a few hours while the hospital staff administered a glucose IV, and my blood sugar returned to normal. Before I was released from the hospital, Pete explained to the doctor that my regular doctor wanted to try for tighter control of my blood sugar in order to avoid the typical long-term consequences. The emergency room doctor explained to Pete in no uncertain terms that if the seizures had continued for a while longer, I could have suffered permanent brain damage or even died. In other words, I had better pay closer attention to short-term consequences or I might not live long enough to suffer any long-term ones. However, even after such a dire warning (which certainly helped to focus my attention), my situation continued to deteriorate.

About once a month I would experience a low I couldn't attribute to anything obvious. The low glucose levels did not seem to be related to insulin levels, food, exercise, stress, or humidity. I definitely noticed the pattern of lows in the log book in which I recorded all my glucose levels and anything out of the ordinary. Eventually, I began to notice a pattern of lows that occurred just before I began to menstruate when my hormonal levels changed. Once the pattern became obvious, I knew what to expect each month

So, diabetes turned me—and my doctors—into investigators. We had explored many of the obvious things that would cause my blood sugar to drop so drastically and quickly, but we were not able to pinpoint the reason in every instance. In an attempt to find out exactly what was happening with my body, and what caused all the lows, my HMO internist thought it might be wise to explore just how fast my stomach was emptying. She thought that possibly I was not getting the full benefit of food if it left my stomach too fast or stayed in too long. She suspected that I might have gastroparesis, which is a form of neuropathy (a medical term for nerve damage) that affects the stomach. Digestion of food may be incomplete or delayed, resulting in nausea, vomiting, or bloating, making blood glucose control difficult. I was not exhibiting any of the typical symptoms, but she wanted to rule out the possibility. To find out, she sent me to a radiologist for a special test. To prepare for the test, I had to eat a fried egg sandwich, which has never been a favorite food of mine because I just can't stomach the crispy edges. To make matters even worse, they used the tasteless bread I call "white sponge bread." When I suggested they offer something a bit more appetizing, that idea was immediately vetoed. Well, I thought, they might really get to see how fast my stomach would empty if I threw up. I did force myself to eat the sandwich—and not throw up. They had coated the food with a radioactive substance that showed up on a screen. The image of the food moving around my stomach fascinated me, but the result of this assessment was that my stomach emptied at a normal rate.

Ryan's delivery

During out first eight years of marriage, Pete and I discussed the possibility of having children. In addition to the questions every person faces about readiness for children such as their financial situation, lifestyle changes, and many others, we also had to answer some very specific questions related to diabetes. Primarily, we wanted to know the likelihood that our child would have diabetes, how the pregnancy would affect my diabetes, and how the diabetes might affect my pregnancy and unborn child. We sought information from a geneticist about the heredity question. This was in 1978. Research, at that time, had not yet firmly established that diabetes was an autoimmune disease. The thinking was that a hereditary factor did increase the risk of the disease but they were not sure why the islet cells in the pancreas were destroyed. Some credence was given to the theory that the insulin producing cells in the pancreas were destroyed by a virus. We were advised that our child may be more likely than the general population to have the disease but the risk was not extremely high. I consulted with my internist as well. I was advised that a pregnancy would require that my diabetes be more closely followed with more office visits to monitor my blood sugars and more frequent urine sugars at home. A pregnancy would increase the demands on my body and I would essentially have to manage the glucose levels for two people. Pete and I discussed all the pros and cons of the situation and decided that the pros definitely outweighed the cons. Shortly after that we were in the midst of a job change and a move, so we waited until we were settled in our new location before I conceived.

I became pregnant with our son Ryan in September of 1980. We were living in a small town in West Virginia. There were two general practitioners in town, but no obstetricians. I called an obstetrician in Cumberland, Maryland—the nearest "big town"—and asked if he had any experience with diabetes and pregnancy. Luckily, he told me he had treated many women with diabetes. So, I set off for the first of many appointments. Cumberland was about an hour's drive away, but we didn't have the option of being treated by anyone closer. The hospital in our town was very small and did not deliver babies, and we hoped we could make it to

Cumberland in time for the delivery. According to the doctor's calculations, my due date was July 5.

Throughout my pregnancy I experienced a few minor reactions when my blood sugar would drop. I would become very sweaty and my vision would blur. These reactions usually occurred with exercise—running at the beginning of the pregnancy, and also cross county skiing. This was before I had a blood glucose meter, so urine testing was my only indicator of high blood sugars and the only means of self monitoring available. I was still taking NPH insulin and I would slightly increase my dose if I found I was spilling sugar. I had my fasting glucose levels taken periodically at the local laboratory, and they were within acceptable ranges. This was before the days when A1c levels were taken; at least they were not available in our area. The A1c is a test that measures a person's average blood glucose level over the past 2 to 3 months. Hemoglobin is the part of a red blood cell that carries oxygen to the body and sometimes hemoglobin joins with the glucose in the bloodstream. Also called hemoglobin A1c (or Hgb A1c), the test is a measure of how much glucose is stuck to the red blood cells, which is proportional to the amount of glucose in the blood over the life of the red blood cell. The test affords a more accurate measure of the blood sugar levels over time compared to daily monitoring with a meter.

I had frequent blood levels drawn at the local hospital and at the end of May my doctor thought that I was possibly experiencing pre-eclampsia or pregnancy induced toxemia. The major symptom was edema (or swelling) of the ankles.

I drove to Cumberland for an appointment with the doctor after he had received the latest blood test result. He told me that because of the high-risk nature of my pregnancy, the unpredictability of my blood sugars, the stress on my body, and my elevated blood level (with the edema), they were going to try to induce labor the next day. They released me from the hospital to have dinner with Pete. My husband and I went out for our last "childless" dinner together. The next day, the doctors told me that they felt the baby had reached a good size and would be okay. This happened on May 30, five weeks before the due date. It was also my birthday!

Hospital staff members started a drip to induce labor and I did have minor contractions. A fetal monitor indicated that the baby was doing well. After several hours, my doctor discussed a Caesarian delivery with us, and we decided to move forward with that option. While they rolled me in to the operating room, I started to feel very shaky and sweaty. I wondered if this was just excitement, or if it was a reaction. As we moved down the hall, I announced that they had to stop. I was having a reaction and needed something to eat. They patiently waited while I drank some juice and ate a cracker. That did the trick, and my roll to the delivery room continued.

Ryan weighed over seven pounds and was born five weeks premature. If I had carried him to full term, we might have needed to consider the name "Mack," as in Mack Truck. Despite Ryan's size, his lungs were not fully developed. He needed to be transferred to a neonatal intensive care unit (NICU). The closest one was three hours away in Morgantown, West Virginia (where my sister Patty lived). Just gaining consciousness after the anesthetic, I caught a brief glimpse of Ryan before they whisked him away.

Pete went to see Ryan during the period when I was recovering and not allowed to travel. My sister had been giving him tender loving care in our absence. He remained in the NICU on oxygen for a week until his lungs could sustain him. Then he was transferred to a "step-down unit." We traveled to Morgantown to be with our new son and take him home when he was 12 days old. I always tell Ryan that he was the best birthday present I ever received.

"The Look"

Over the years, Ryan and Pete became attuned to changes in my body language and facial expression when my blood sugar started to drop. I acquired, what my husband and son would describe as "The Look"—a vacant, not totally focused, dull kind of appearance. Once when I was talking to my son, he said, "Mom, you have 'The Look.' Better check your blood sugar." I denied that I was having a reaction, and rushed to the mirror to see for myself what "The Look" looked like. To me, I looked normal. But just to appease him, I agreed to take my blood sugar. It registered at 26, an extremely low number. Below 70 is considered an insulin reaction. Because my brain was not getting the sugar it needed to function, I couldn't recognize the symptoms of low blood sugar.

Biking

One very warm Sunday in January of 1991, I decided to take advantage of the good weather and ride my bike four miles to meet my sister, Paula, so that we could catch a movie matinee. I ate some popcorn at the movie and thought this would suffice until I returned home after the movie. We left the theater at about 4 p.m. Feeling fine, I jumped on my bike and started heading home. The temperature had dropped while I was watching the movie and the sun was starting to go down. My body had to work a little harder to produce enough heat to keep me warm, and I was thus using more energy. I remember reaching the top of a hill and zipping up my jacket. The next thing I remember was waking up in the intensive care unit of a hospital several days later. My family filled me in on the part of my life I had missed.

Apparently I had ridden part way down the hill when my blood sugar dropped drastically and immediately. My momentum kept me going even though I had lost consciousness. At the bottom of the hill, I must have slowed down, fallen over, and hit the curb. A passerby saw me lying motionless, and ran to a nearby house to get help. They called 911, and I was taken to the hospital. In the meantime, I was late for dinner, so my husband called Paula, but she could only say when we left the theater. At some point that evening, they tell me I regained consciousness enough to tell hospital staffers my name and my sister's telephone number. One of my many mistakes that day was to leave the house without identification. I had simply put enough money in my pocket to cover the movie and popcorn. Another grave mistake was that I had no medic alert information on me. Hospital personnel would have been able to call my husband earlier and they also would have been able to take corrective measures to relieve my hypoglycemia. It was obvious that I was unconscious but one of the contributing factors to that was the hypoglycemia in addition to a concussion.

After a social worker from the hospital called Paula, she asked whether they realized that I had diabetes. The social worker dropped the phone, and yelled down the hall to deliver that bit of news. Afterwards, Paula called Pete to tell him what she knew. Then the social worker called Pete to relate my whereabouts and my condition. I had sustained a concussion (I wasn't wearing a helmet), a broken

43

collarbone, and many broken ribs. During three days of slipping in and out of consciousness in the intensive care unit, I don't remember Pete or most of my other visitors, but I had one lucid flash. I remember talking to my brother-in-law, Tom, who was wearing a bright maroon and gold sweater. I can't remember anything else. As I started to recover, I graduated to a regular room, and remained in the hospital for a total of 10 days before going home.

We ordered a special hospital bed for our house, so I could sit up without having to change positions. We put the bed in the downstairs bedroom to eliminate the problem the stairs posed. Making slow, steady progress, I was eventually able to get up out of bed. Within a few weeks, I reached the point when I could walk around the block. My husband was between jobs, so he became my nurse and provided encouragement and support throughout my ordeal. Eleven weeks after the accident, I finally returned to work.

When the bike incident occurred, I was not wearing a helmet or a medical alert bracelet and carried no identification. Since then, I always carry identification, even if I am just walking to the mailbox and I always wear a helmet when riding my bike. My medical alert bracelet became a part of my body which I did not remove until after the transplant. My bicycle accident was a very tough way for me to learn those lessons, and I hope that others with diabetes can learn from my experience.

Snorkeling

During a December 1997 trip to the Turks and Caicos Islands, my husband and I were snorkeling off the coast of Grand Turk. We had ventured quite a distance from shore and had been in the water for about 45 minutes. I had eaten lunch, so I thought I would be okay for a while. However, I started having a lot of difficulty coordinating the use of my mask and mouthpiece. Taking off the mask and dipping it in the water to clear the lens, I tried again and again to make it fit without leaking. My husband asked me what was wrong. He watched me for a brief period and said, "Ellen, you're having a reaction." Of course, I belligerently denied it. I was wearing a waterproof container around my neck usually used to protect money and keys while swimming. In mine, thank goodness, I had a roll of LifeSavers. I was not able to get to the candy so Pete struggled to get the case off, open it, and make me eat the candy. This all happened while he was treading water and supporting me. After I ate the candy, Pete hauled me in using the sidestroke method he had learned in lifesaving class when he was a teenager. He moved me in to shallow water where I could stand. This wasn't easy, because I'm only 5 feet 2 inches tall. Finally, I started to recover as I ate more candy. At last I could touch the bottom and walked out on my own.

The birth of Eileen

In November of 1996, my sister Paula was due to deliver her third child. Her husband and I were her coaches, and we each had a beeper from the hospital so that we'd know when it was time to assist with the delivery. I had helped them deliver their first two children. Paula and Tom lived about an hour away, and they had assured me that I could make it in time for the birth.

After walking about a mile to a class at Kaiser (my HMO) one blustery evening when Paula was due at any moment, I took a seat and soon realized I was missing part of what the speaker was saying. Although I thought he was just a boring speaker and not able to hold my attention, I was actually drifting in and out of consciousness. By the end of the class, I was totally unconscious. My husband informed me later that, at first, the teacher thought I had fallen asleep in class, but had quickly realized the gravity of the situation.

HMO staff members took me down to the urgent care section of the same building, and thanks to my medic alert bracelet and a pen I had with my name on it, the staff immediately figured out the proper treatment. A glucose IV brought me back to consciousness. After my husband arrived and I regained enough awareness to ask questions, he told me that my sister had beeped me during my episode, and that she had given birth to a girl. My disappointment in missing the birth was overwhelming. I was very angry with myself. Apparently the cold temperature, the stress of anticipating the birth, and the exercise of walking had caused my blood sugar to plummet.

The next morning I drove to the hospital to visit my beautiful new niece, Eileen. My sister was very understanding when I apologized for having missed the birth, and we hugged and cried.

Driving on the Beltway

NPH insulin, the time-released insulin that I was taking, usually peaked for me about nine hours after I had taken it. This meant that it peaked at around 4 p.m., when I was driving home from work. On one particular afternoon, things had gone according to plan all day. I had taken my normal amount of insulin, eaten my regular lunch, and walked my usual half hour after lunch. I didn't experience any unusual stressors at work. In fact, everything seemed normal. But while driving home, I realized that I didn't know where I was. I felt confused, and wasn't sure which exit I should take to get off the Capital Beltway. The Beltway is an eight lane interstate highway that passes near our home—not unfamiliar territory to me.

I had driven the same route every workday for fifteen years. I knew enough to pull off the road and I stopped on the shoulder. My candy was right next to me, but my brain was not functioning well enough to allow me to get it. I immediately lost consciousness and slumped over the wheel. When I returned to the real world, I was lying in the back of an ambulance with a glucose IV in my arm. The paramedics took me to the hospital because my blood sugar was still dangerously low, even though the IV had been pumping the sugar solution into my body. By the time we got to the hospital, I felt fine and had regained my senses. Of course, I had to remain for a few more hours to get clearance from a doctor before I was allowed to leave. On the way to the hospital, one of the paramedics had called my husband at work, told him that they had me in the back of the ambulance, and told him our destination. Later, Pete came to pick me up and, on our way to ransom my car from the lot where it had been towed, he said that it had been difficult to get any work done after receiving the call.

Aerobics

For almost ten years I have taken a twice-weekly dance aerobics class at a neighborhood elementary school. Diane has been my instructor for all those years, and we have become friends. She and everyone else in the class knew I had diabetes. The steps and routines have become very familiar, but on two separate occasions I had great difficulty following what was going on. I continually missed steps and went the wrong way, falling behind the rest of the class. This was very unusual behavior for me. On one occasion, a friend in the class stopped me and insisted that I eat my candy, which I always carry with me. On the second occasion, my blood sugar once again dropped and I fell over the hypoglycemic cliff before I even knew I was on the edge. By the time I regained consciousness, Diane had called my husband and forced me to eat my candy. On each of those occasions I had taken my blood sugar before the class and it had been within the target range. For reasons we don't know, on those nights it dropped too far.

On April 15, 1999, I had done well in class with no indication that my blood sugar was dropping. While walking out of the building I had a normal conversation with Diane and started to drive home along my customary route, a distance of only eight blocks. I made a turn on to what I thought was my street, stopped the car in front of what I thought was my house and then lost consciousness. In fact, I was two blocks from home. The top on my convertible was down so it was easy for people passing by to see into the car. A man on his way to the mailbox with his tax return noticed something strange about the car parked in the middle of the street with the driver leaning over the wheel. He approached and asked if I was okay. He says that I did respond to him, but that he could not understand what I said, although he was able to surmise that the real answer to his question was a resounding "NO." He immediately called 911. The police and paramedics came, found identification with my address. The policeman went to my home and brought my husband back to the scene. When he arrived, the paramedics were treating me in the back of the ambulance with a glucose IV. This brought me back to consciousness and I recovered enough so they could take me home. Pete drove the two blocks in my car. I had been sweating profusely and he got soaked sitting in my driver's seat. Because I had identification and a medic alert bracelet the situation was brought under control much more quickly than it might have been otherwise.

Three hours later

Another trip over the hypoglycemic cliff caused me to lose consciousness while driving during my workday. As a part of my job, I visit the homes of preschool children to administer educational testing that will help determine if they are eligible for special education programs in the public school system. One morning, I left my office at 8:45 a.m. for a 9:30 appointment. At 10:00, the mother of the child I was to visit called my office wondering why I had not yet arrived. Knowing my history, my colleagues became suspicious about what might have happened. They called the police and told them I was missing. The police offered suggestions about where I might have gone, possibly shopping or visiting. My officemates emphasized that this was a medical emergency. Police officers were dispatched to the home I was supposed to visit, and they waited for me to arrive—for three hours. My colleagues had called my husband to tell him that I was missing. One police officer called my husband three times over the next few hours to learn background information, to ask where he thought I might be, and to get help in completing his paperwork.

Meanwhile, I had taken a wrong turn onto a dead end street. At the end, I stopped the car because I simply did not know what else to do. I must have been slipping toward unconsciousness. I remember turning off the engine, then I must have slumped over the steering wheel, and once again fell over the crumbling edge of the hypoglycemic cliff. My candy was within reach, but I could not get it. Much later, I regained consciousness. One theory that my doctor proposed was that my liver finally kicked in and produced enough sugar to revive me. After I ate some candy, I began to feel better and was competent enough to drive. After going a short distance, I was able to orient myself and realized I was only about 10 minutes away from the office. It was now close to 12:00. I had been missing for three hours!

My arrival at the office caused great sighs of relief. Yet there was an undercurrent of resentment and anger that something like this had happened again. I was also frustrated. The disease was becoming extremely frightening and increasingly out of my control. I began to feel powerless despite all my efforts to stay in control. My condition was becoming potentially life threatening for both myself and others.

My colleagues

At work my colleagues became experts at sensing my blood sugar levels. They often had to check on me to see if I was OK. My desk sat in the back of the room, and my friends would often stop by to make sure I was still conscious. They had learned to do this because quite a few times they had stopped by and found that I was "not at home," so to speak. Sitting at my desk, I would be covered with sweat and not able to answer their questions. A few times I had lost consciousness and they had called 911. When I would regain my senses, the emergency medical technicians would say, "Oh, hi Ellen, we're here again." It's not a good sign when the paramedics know you by name.

Zero reading

After one of my falls over the hypoglycemic cliff I had been given a bottle of Gatorade in an effort to bring to me back to consciousness. The emergency medical technicians were taking my blood sugar to make sure it had returned to a normal range. Susan, a friend and coworker who has diabetes, asked what my blood sugar was. The technician was hesitant to tell her. She explained that she would understand the number because she had diabetes. He said that there must be something wrong with his meter because the reading was zero. He tested my blood sugar again and it was once again a big fat zero. Although I had regained consciousness enough to drink normally, I do not remember anything about the incident. Shortly after that my glucose level began to return to a normal range.

Alarming frequency and intensity

After living with diabetes for approximately thirty-five years I started to have reactions that required assistance from others. I lost the ability to sense these reactions, and was unable to take action to stop my blood sugar from dropping. I found myself on the crumbling edge of the hypoglycemic cliff more and more often.

The intensity of my reactions varied greatly and fell along a continuum. My husband, Pete, and I divided this continuum into three general categories, or levels, based on my level of functioning and the intervention required.

In the least severe reactions, what we called Level-1, I was sometimes able to answer Pete's questions but my response time was slower than normal. I did not recognize that I had to eat to increase my blood sugar level. I was able to follow directions and control my actions during a Level-1 reaction so Pete would encourage me to eat something. Frequently, I would eat but sometimes, as my blood sugar dropped, I became positively obstinate and would adamantly deny that I was having a reaction. There were a few times when Pete noticed some early signs and said that I was starting to have a reaction, but I felt fine and seemed to be able to function quite well. In those cases, he challenged me to take my blood sugar and said that if it was low then I would have to eat. I agreed just to prove to him that I was okay. Of course, most of the time he was right, and I had to eat.

During Level-2 reactions, I was conscious but not able to do anything for myself, so Pete had to feed me. He would either put LifeSavers candy into my mouth—if I could chew, or he squeezed a tube of glucose solution into my mouth. This solution was very sweet and similar to cake frosting. Sometimes I would go into a reaction at the dinner table, and then Pete would try to give me spoonfuls of whatever was on my plate. When I started to show signs of a reaction, Pete would try to gauge the severity by doing a mental status exam to assess whether I was oriented to time, place, and person (he used to be a psychologist). He would start by asking my name, and the names of our son and other relatives. The day of the week, month, and season would follow. Our address, city, and state would be next. Pete would then check my short-term memory with questions about recent activities such as what we had done that day. In the midst of a hypoglycemic reaction, I would struggle to respond to his questions and truly have to search within the depths of my mind to find the correct answers. I could almost always say my own name, but my answers to the other questions varied a lot. According to Pete, they helped him to gauge the required amount and type of intervention. Also, as I came out of a reaction, my responses helped him to figure out when to stop feeding me.

The most severe reactions, Level-3, required a shot of glucagon after I had lost consciousness. Level-3 reactions were rare, but followed a consistent pattern. Pete recalls being awakened at four a.m. from a deep sleep. He remembers hearing my uneven breathing patterns and unusual vocalizations, which progressed to grand mal seizures and unconsciousness before he could feed me. He would then resort to using glucagon. Glucagon comes as two separate solutions, one in a syringe, and the other in a separate vial. The solution in the syringe needs to be injected into the vial, gently mixed and then drawn back slowly into the syringe and injected into the person having the reaction. Pete followed these directions while I was seizing, moaning, groaning, and writhing all over the bed covered with sweat. It was an effort for him to get me still enough to administer the injection. He would roll me on my side; sit on my hip bone, facing my feet so that my flailing arms would not knock the syringe out of his hand. These were very stressful situations for him both emotionally and physically.

It usually took about 10 minutes for the glucagon to take full effect and bring my blood sugar back to a normal level. As I showed signs of recovery, Pete would ask questions to determine my progress. I would slowly return to consciousness and struggle to respond. It was similar to what I imagine drowning must be like. I wanted desperately to return to the surface but it took a supreme effort to get there. It would have been so much easier to just relax and fall back into unconsciousness but I knew I just could not do that. I could hear and understand what he was saying but I just could not formulate the words to answer. I would gradually return to an alert state and then the realization would dawn on me that I had once again had a severe reaction. Heaving an enormous sigh, I would vow that this would not happen again.

I was desperate to find a way to prevent these reactions, but I was becoming less and less successful. I would analyze everything I did while trying to determine what caused me to crash. Something new always popped up that I hadn't accounted for, and that would once again cause me to fall over the cliff. During his career, Pete has been a psychologist, a computer programmer, and a systems analyst. He helped me greatly in trying to analyze all my data. We made lists with all the factors we could think of that could influence my blood sugars, trying to predict and prevent reactions. After each reaction we would add more data. One surprising factor we were able to determine from this analysis was the wind, which could be a major factor even when it was 55 degrees and sunny. I learned to protect myself more diligently from the wind chill which would cause my blood sugar to drop.

I am eternally grateful to my family and friends for all their support. They were always there when I needed them.

Chapter 4
ELIGIBILITY

In June of 2000, doctors conducting medical research in Edmonton, Canada, published the results of an exciting new procedure that held great promise for treating Type 1 diabetes, and which might possibly be the long awaited cure. It was published in The New England Journal of Medicine, other medical media, and the general press. Doctors James Shapiro, Jonathan Lakey, Ray Rajotte, and their colleagues had experimented with a procedure to transplant "islets of Langerhans" from the pancreas of a donor into the liver of a person with diabetes. The Edmonton team modified the previous protocol to overcome shortcomings that were felt to have limited the success of earlier islet transplant attempts. Most importantly, they decided to transplant more islets; they decided to transplant islets from more than one donor for each recipient. They also transplanted the islets immediately after they were isolated as opposed to keeping them in tissue culture for a day or two. Another change was that they avoided steroids in the immunosuppressive regimen. The studies, conducted in Edmonton and published in 2000, reported that 7 patients had received transplanted islets, and that all were insulin free a year later. This was a phenomenal and unprecedented success. Researchers had been attempting to transplant islet cells for thirty years before this and had been unsuccessful in achieving such apparently uniform insulin independence. This was extremely promising. I read that, as part of the research, the protocol needed to be repeated with many more subjects and at many more sites. My excitement grew when the replication sites were announced and I realized that the National Institutes of Health was one of the sites. The NIH campus in Bethesda, Maryland, is very close to my home—only twenty-one minutes door to door.

I found a Web site called www.clinicaltrials.gov that listed the requirements for eligibility. Patients had to meet specific criteria even to be considered for evaluation:

- Have Type 1 diabetes
- The diabetes must be "brittle" (a term used when a person's blood glucose level often moves from low to high and from high to low)
- Be between the ages of eighteen and sixty
- Must not have kidney failure
- Must not have undergone a previous transplant
- Must not have an allergy to iodine or x-ray contrast agents
- Must not have a history of any cancer (including skin cancer)
- Must not be medically obese (defined as a body mass index of 30 kg/m2 or greater)

I mentally checked off each criteria as I read it. In early fall of 2000, I downloaded the application, completed the detailed medical history, and submitted the forms. I checked the mail daily looking for a reply, and each time I sighed with disappointment. In November, I finally received the letter that invited me to start the process to determine if I was eligible for the study.

The very first step in this process was an interview with Dr. David Harlan, the lead investigator, and his team. The team included a nurse coordinator named Lisa Viviano, and a research fellow, Dr. Boaz Hirshberg. Dr. Harlan started the interview by saying he was going to try to talk me out of this procedure. He is extremely concerned about the safety of this protocol for his patients. He very carefully detailed all the steps involved in the process, from eligibility to the actual transplant procedure and the follow-up. He explained the risks, and especially emphasized the experimental nature of the procedure. No long-term data were available yet. He gave me a consent form (actually it was more like 8 or 9 pages) detailing the procedure, the risks, and the treatment after the procedure. He asked me to take it home and study it. I discussed the document with my husband line by line and word by word. The consent form stated that participating in NIH experiments was entirely voluntary and that I could choose to not take part or withdraw at any time. The introduction stated that that there may be no benefit to me. They were clearly not guaranteeing anything. The primary purpose was research. The specific objective was to test whether the promising results achieved in Edmonton, Canada could be replicated at NIH. The study consisted of three parts, a screening evaluation, a treatment phase, and a follow-up phase. The document also detailed the side effects and risks involved. These included, as specified in the protocol:

- Risks associated with the procedure itself. The islets are infused into the portal vein, which leads to the liver where the islets remain. As such, the procedure was associated with the danger of bleeding, infection, and damage to the liver, gall bladder, or to the blood vessels within the liver, including blood clotting within the blood vessel where the islets were to be infused. Any of these complications could be sufficiently severe to cause death.

- Risk of infection. Immunosuppressive drugs are given to prevent rejection. Because the immune system is suppressed, there is a risk of developing serious infections and certain cancers.

- Risk of a body becoming "educated" to reject organs in the future. That is, by receiving transplanted islets, my body's immune system would learn to recognize the tissue from the islet donor. If I ever needed another transplant (say a kidney transplant should my kidneys fail), my previous islet transplant could make it more difficult to find a suitable donor. My body's immune system would be "educated" to recognize donor tissues, which might make it more difficult for me to qualify for a future transplant.

The drugs used to prevent rejection have known side effects. These included high blood pressure, increased cholesterol levels, impaired kidney function, impaired ability to make red blood cells, and other side effects. Each person's individual tolerance to the drugs is different, and the side effects vary widely.

After writing down all of our questions, I returned to NIH, and Dr. Harlan addressed all of them. Many of our questions concerned the success rates and experiences of patients that had already had the transplant. I was curious about what my chances were and how long the wait might be. Some questions concerned the side effects of the immunosuppressive drugs and the treatment for those effects. We wanted to know how long the transplant would last and what the long-term prognosis was. Unfortunately, Dr. Harlan did not have definite answers to all our questions because the treatment was still experimental. At this point in my life

I was desperate to find a solution to my hypoglycemia unawareness, and nothing else seemed to be available for me. I was extremely hopefully that this treatment might be the solution to my problem. I signed the consent in early November of 2000, and officially began the eligibility process.

The testing was very detailed and involved. From November to February, I spent many days at NIH using up all of my accumulated sick leave without ever being really "sick." The National Institutes of Health is located in Bethesda, Maryland. It is a sprawling campus of more than 50 buildings on 23 acres that is nestled in a residential neighborhood. The NIH consists of 27 institutes, the Library of Medicine, and the Office of the Director. There are also seven centers located on the campus where 18,000 people are employed. Many paths wander among the buildings and the trees, creating a university campus feeling. The Clinical Center, Building 10, where the NIDDK (National Institute of Diabetes, and Digestive and Kidney Diseases) is located is an imposing 14 story red brick building with a labyrinth of hallways and stairs that extend for an impressive 29 miles. A unique inner physical structure assures that research laboratories are located close to the patients. This allows a scientist to work in both the lab and the clinic.

My team wanted to make sure that I had all my body parts and that they all worked. They wanted to ensure that their data would be clean, and not tainted by any unknown conditions or complications. And most important, they wanted to make sure that the experimental procedure would not place me at any undue risk due to some silent medical condition. My nurse coordinator, Lisa, was in charge of making appointments in the specialty departments.

A cardiologist evaluated my heart function. An echocardiogram, electrocardiogram (EKG) and a thallium stress test were part of that evaluation. The echocardiogram allowed me to see the chambers of my heart open and close on the monitor near the exam table. It was fascinating to see my heart in operation. Another part of the heart assessment included a thallium stress test. I looked forward to this assessment, since I would get to exercise. As I started the procedure, the technician asked if I had taken a pregnancy test. There would be a possible danger to a fetus because of the use of radiation in the procedure. I wasn't worried about that possibility, since my last menstrual cycle had been twelve months earlier and I was fifty-two years old. But, we had to wait to start the stress test until the team received the results of a rush pregnancy test. The results came back negative, so we could proceed. I felt and looked like the bionic woman as I started to run on the treadmill with many wires attached to my body. One of the lines was infusing a thallium solution. That would allow the x-ray technician to trace the path of my blood through my circulatory system after I completed the exercise portion. A monitor displayed my heart rate as I started to move. I exercise frequently and am in fairly good aerobic condition. Nina, the technician, kept a close eye on the monitors as the time ticked away. She commented that it usually didn't take that long to elevate a person's heart rate to the upper limits required for the test. After I finally reached the upper limit required, I was wheeled to the radiology suite, where the team traced the flow of my blood after exercise. They didn't note any difficulties with my heart or circulation.

Another requirement for eligibility was that the islets in my pancreas had to produce no insulin. I learned from my NIH team that a surprising number of people with Type 1 diabetes, even people who have had the disease most of their lives, and had been taking insulin, still produce small amounts of insulin. While such individuals don't make nearly enough insulin for them to maintain normal blood sugar levels (and thus they must inject insulin), the medical researchers wanted to make sure that only the islets they infused produced the insulin required to make me independent of insulin injections. In other words, the NIH team wanted to know that any insulin they measured in my blood stream after my transplant had to come from the cells they transplanted, and not from my own pancreas. Their testing required that I undergo an assessment called an arginine stimulated c-peptide test, which is a timed measurement using two intravenous lines, one for deposits the other for withdrawals. Arginine is part of the food that we eat but the NIH team gives it in a highly concentrated form in an injected solution. This causes the body to produce insulin. Blood is withdrawn at timed intervals for ten minutes. Connecting peptide (c-peptide) is a substance the pancreas releases into the bloodstream in amounts that are equal to the insulin produced. By measuring C-peptide levels, the doctors can assess how much insulin the body is making. This is true even in patients still injecting insulin (since injected insulin does not contain c-peptide; only insulin made in the body is made with the c-peptide). The results of my initial arginine test indicated that my pancreas was not producing any insulin. I had successfully completed another step in the eligibility process.

On other visits to the radiology department, they conducted other tests. An abdominal ultrasound made sure that my gall bladder, liver, and liver blood vessel anatomy was normal. The team used a twenty-four hour urine sample to assess whether my kidneys were functioning normally. I collected my urine for a twenty-four period, and they tested to see if any protein was present in it, and also to measure how much creatinine I was excreting. Creatinine is a waste product from protein in the diet and from the muscles of the body. It is removed from the body by the kidneys. The kidneys do not normally filter protein, but when the kidneys are damaged by diabetes, protein is found in the urine. All of my organs were working well, and I moved on to the next step.

I donated what seemed like gallons of blood to the phlebotomy department. All the technicians knew me by name. My veins are very small, and difficult to locate. They often rolled out of the way or collapsed during a blood draw. I was grateful that the people at phlebotomy were very friendly and caring, and did not even cringe when they saw me coming. Otherwise, I might have dreaded that part.

I was scheduled for a flexible sigmoidoscopy, which enables the physician to look at the inside of the large intestine from the rectum through the last part of the colon, called the sigmoid, or descending, colon. With flexible sigmoidoscopy, the physician can see sites of bleeding, inflammation, abnormal growths, and ulcers in the descending colon and rectum. The team explained specific requirements of what to eat and not eat for a few days before my appointment. When I returned on the day of the appointment, the technician asked if I had followed all the recommendations and I responded positively. Then he asked if I had completed the enema. "What enema?" I asked. I had forgotten to pick up the enema kit from the pharmacy on my last visit. So I had to start all over again. We scheduled another appointment, and everything went according to plan the next time. The results indicated that everything was within normal limits. During another internal exploration the doctors used a lighted exploratory tube to view the twists and turns in the depths of my intestines. They were looking for any abnormalities, and thankfully they didn't find any.

I also had a bone scan to check for osteoporosis. The spidery, black and white picture produced by the scan looked like a Halloween decoration or a party favor. Luckily, the results indicated normal bone density.

Another specialty department I visited was ophthalmology. They examined my eyes with intense lights, and measured the fluid pressure inside the eye. Since 1993, I have had glaucoma, a condition where the pressure inside the eye increases and can lead to blindness. I place drops into my eyes twice daily to reduce the pressure. I developed cataracts in both eyes after my diabetes was misdiagnosed as the "flu" for many months. The staff members in the ophthalmology department at NIH were very interested in my eyes and took many photographs of them. They did note a little bit of background retinopathy in the back of my eyes. Background retinopathy is a type of damage to the retina of the eye marked by bleeding, fluid accumulation and abnormal dilation of the blood vessels. Background retinopathy is an early stage of diabetic retinopathy. It is also called simple or nonproliferative retinopathy. Retinopathy is damage to the retina—the light-sensitive area at the back of the eye—and the blood vessels serving it. They kept asking me if I was sure I had diabetes for 40 years. Yes, I was very sure of that fact, I told them. They were amazed that my eyes did not show more damage.

The team also scheduled a personal interview with the social worker to assess how comfortable I was with the whole procedure. The social worker was most interested in my support network. My family and friends who had rescued me so many times in the past were very encouraging in my efforts to explore this clinical trial. They also hoped that I would no longer become unconscious without warning. The social worker also discussed the time commitment involved in the whole trial, including the actual transplant procedure, the collection of extensive data, frequent drug level checks, lab procedures, and many outpatient visits to NIH. In addition, they were trying to determine if I would be able to understand and follow the complex medical regimen required after transplant. Understanding that there was no guarantee of success was another component that was essential on my part.

A final interview with the team was arranged, and again Dr. Harlan reviewed the whole procedure. He told me that results of all the eligibility procedures indicated that I was a good candidate and met all the requirements. And again, he stressed the experimental nature of the project. He informed me that I was free to drop out of the protocol any time I wished, and that the decision was entirely mine to make. My only hesitation, and it was slight, involved the possible side effect of the immunosuppressive drugs. This was an unknown factor. The literature from the Edmonton project had presented some side effects. But this was all still very new. The limited amount of existing data were from a small number of patients and were only two years old. My team could not predict how my body would react to the drugs. Because of the ever-present hypoglycemia unawareness, I was willing to try it, and signed the consent form once again.

Five others had undergone the procedure at NIH before I did. One person had received only one transplant because of a complication during the procedure, and she remained on insulin but her dosage dropped. Three of the patients were totally insulin free, and the fifth had much better control of her disease with a greatly reduced amount of insulin. All five had previously suffered from hypoglycemia unawareness and after transplant; they no longer had this condition. That was even more encouraging.

64

Chapter 5
LISTED

There were risks involved in the procedure, and my signature on the permission form indicated that I had given my "informed consent." The doctors had explained the possible complications on at least four separate occasions. Possible problems included increased difficulty finding a suitable kidney donor if that ever became necessary, bleeding during the transplant, infection, and side effects of the immunosuppressive drugs that I would take for the rest of my life (or at least as long as my transplanted islets made insulin). With all these things in mind, I was still willing to go ahead with the transplant.

Would the procedure work? I had no way of knowing the answer, but I was becoming desperate to find a solution to an increasingly life-threatening situation. If it didn't work, heart problems, blindness, amputation, and kidney failure might be in my future. The possible immediate consequences of problems related to diabetes were much more dire—death. The ever-present danger of hypoglycemia unawareness put not only me but also others in grave danger. Sudden unconsciousness put me at an ever-present risk that this might result in injury to me, or even death. The possibility of a car accident involving others also loomed dangerously near. It was extremely frightening to not have control over when these incidents might occur.

In late February of 2001, I got the call from Lisa stating that I was officially listed. This meant that I could be called whenever NIH received a pancreas from a donor with a matching blood type. This was great, exciting news. Reminding Lisa that it was only 21 minutes from my home to NIH, I knew I could be there quickly. It would take the lab six hours to isolate the donor islet cells and prepare them for transplant. I was ready. At this point, I broke down and purchased a cell phone so I wouldn't miss the all-important call. Previous to this point I had felt that a person trying to get in touch with me, could leave a message and I would get back to them when it was convenient. No call was that important up until this point!

I had to send blood to NIH every two weeks. A nurse at my HMO would draw the blood, and I would mail the package to NIH. They wanted to make sure nothing unusual was happening in my body, so they needed current information on hand to be prepared when a donor pancreas arrived.

I quickly learned how to communicate with the team at NIH even in extraordinary situations. My husband and I had planned a ski trip to Canada in early January. One evening shortly before our scheduled departure, I had just finished an aerobic workout at home and was stretching. A sudden, intense pain in my knee made it very difficult even to walk. Even after x-rays, my orthopedic doctor, Dr. Sidney Chetta could only explain what had happened as "an event." I used a cane for few weeks and went back to the physical therapy office where I had spent many months the year before when I broke my wrist. They all warmly welcomed me back. My cane was decorated with a horn, rear view mirror, and colorful tape—my attempt to make something unpleasant a little more tolerable.

Dr. Chetta suggested postponing the ski trip to March, which we did. I faithfully performed the exercises prescribed by my physical therapist and was ready to go by mid-March. I informed my team at NIH that I would be unavailable for a week while we went skiing in Banff, Canada. We had a wonderful time and I returned with all my body parts intact. I was able to carry my meter and an insulin pen with me while skiing and make adjustments as necessary for exercise. I am proud to say I had no reactions while skiing.

No matter where I was, my NIH team wanted to know exactly what was happening with my blood sugars throughout the day and night. Using the carbohydrate system of food calculation, I recorded how many carbohydrates I ate at each meal and took a shot with a corresponding amount of fast-acting insulin. I measured my blood sugar before every meal, two hours after each meal and once at three a.m. Because of my recent history of severe hypoglycemic reactions while driving, I also took my blood sugar before starting the car. We were attempting to fine-tune a very complicated system. Things were definitely improving, but I continued to experience reactions and high blood sugar levels. The range between my highs and lows continued to be significant. Communicating data to NIH allowed the doctors to respond every day with advice and adjustments.

Chapter 6
THE PUMP

In May 2001, the NIH team decided to try to establish better glycemic control with the resources we had available. The team decided that we should give the pump a try while waiting for the call about a donor. I had not used the pump previously because I had been waiting for the advancement of the closed loop system, which doctors had promised would be coming soon. The closed system refers to a pump, or an insulin delivery system, and a glucometer, or a blood glucose meter, all working as one system. This system is often referred to as an artificial pancreas. Unfortunately, at that point it was not ready yet (and it is still not ready). I was desperate to eliminate falls over the hypoglycemic cliff, so I agreed to try the pump by itself.

A representative from the pump company and my transplant coordinator met me for a training session at four o'clock in the afternoon. NPH insulin reaches its peak about this time, and I thought my blood sugar would drop. Sure enough, during the training, I started to experience a low. I listened to what the representative was saying and nodded in all the appropriate places, but I eventually realized that I was just not processing what she was saying and it was not making sense. I put a quick halt to everything by announcing the reaction, and we stopped so I could eat something. My reaction, however, caused me to miss a piece of information that would soon become critical. I left the office wearing the pump, and was on my way to what I would hope would be better control and fewer hypoglycemic episodes.

The pump itself is about the size of a deck of cards and is an insulin-delivering device that can be worn on a belt or kept in a pocket. An insulin pump connects to a narrow, flexible plastic tubing that ends with a needle inserted just under the skin. I used the fatty tissue in my midriff. Users set the pump to give a steady trickle or basal amount of insulin continuously throughout the day. The user can trigger the pump to release bolus doses of insulin (several units at a time) at meals and at times when blood glucose is too high, based on the amount of carbohydrates consumed and blood sugar levels. Pump users have to fill each new tube with 20 units of insulin before the pump can deliver the insulin. This process, referred to as "priming the pump" allows it to function properly by ensuring that insulin is available at the needle the first time that it is needed. Users also have to change the tube and insertion point and place a new needle every few days.

Soon it was time for me to change the tube and the insertion point for the first time since the training. Before leaving for work, I made the change and ate breakfast. When I checked my blood sugar at work two hours later, I discovered it was in the 200s—a high level. To mitigate the high level, I gave myself a bolus of a few more units of insulin via the pump. Puzzlement and surprise followed an hour later when I found my blood sugar kept going up instead of down. I pumped a little bit more insulin into the tube each time thinking it was reaching my body.

But to my dismay, my blood sugars were continuing to rise, not fall, escalating into the 300s.

Assuming that something must be wrong with the tubing, I threw the tube away and started all over again. My blood sugars continued to rise into the 400s despite the many additional boluses I pumped into the tube. It was now about eleven o'clock in the morning. I was very nauseous, and started throwing up in the bathroom. While I was sitting on the floor in the stall, a woman entered the bathroom and asked if I was OK. I explained to her shoes that I was very ill, and asked if she would please alert someone in my office to come and assist me. She quickly scurried out of the room, and I could hear her feet run down the hall to my office. My friend Colleen came down and compassionately asked what she could do. When I told her I was considering calling 911, she realized how serious the situation was. She called NIH and explained the details to them. They wanted to see me right away. Since I was in no condition to drive, my colleagues called my husband to pick me up.

We arrived at NIH around two o'clock. Carol, the representative from the pump manufacturer, met us there as well as my doctors and nurse coordinator. They were all anxious to determine what caused me to become so ill. They reviewed with me all the events that had occurred over the past couple of days. I explained all that had happened and described exactly what I had done when changing the pump equipment. Then Carol asked the critical question: "Did you prime the pump?" I smashed my palm against my forehead as I realized I had not primed the pump, and that had caused my problems. In other words, the tube connecting the pump to my body was empty. When I thought I was injecting insulin, I was just injecting air! That was the critical piece of information I missed when I had a reaction during the training session—the pump must be primed so that it can actually deliver the insulin. It was a relief to realize that this problem was easily corrected. We immediately primed the pump, and my blood sugar quickly returned to an acceptable level.

The danger had been that I was having a hyperglycemic episode (high blood glucose) that could have resulted in ketoacidosis. Diabetic ketoacidosis is an emergency condition in which extremely high blood glucose levels, along with a severe lack of insulin, result in the breakdown of body fat for energy and an accumulation of ketone acids in the blood and urine. Signs of DKA are nausea and vomiting, stomach pain, fruity breath odor, and rapid breathing. Untreated DKA can lead to coma and death.

The pump did offer me more freedom and flexibility. Calculating carbohydrates and making proper insulin adjustments got easier as I became more familiar and experienced with the pump. When exercising, I could lower my insulin dose or simply remove the pump. Of course, this all took some practice and more frequent monitoring of my blood sugar levels to keep tabs on the situation. Data collection and contact with the team at NIH helped guide me through the learning process.

The pump did even out my blood sugars. My highs were not as high, and my lows were not as low. However, hypoglycemia unawareness still posed a problem.

(Tip: I used to wear my pump in my bra. I placed it in a baby sock to protect my skin from irritation.)

Chapter 7
THE CALL AND THE TRANSPLANT

On June 13, 2001, while driving home from work on the Beltway, I was listening to a radio talk show program when I heard a phone ringing. "Why don't they answer that phone?" I thought. It just kept ringing and ringing. It finally hit me—my phone was ringing. But then I had to find the phone. Digging around in the bag on the seat next me, I finally grabbed the phone and answered the call, thinking it must be my husband or son.

It was Lisa, my transplant coordinator. They had found a donor for me. He was a male who had died in an accident. They expected the pancreas to arrive within a few hours. It was being flown in to Reagan National Airport and then a courier would deliver it to NIH. Lisa instructed me to go home, have something to eat and then go to NIH. I remained very calm and agreed with all her instructions. After I hung up the phone, I let out a big loud yelp. People in the cars around me probably were wondering what radio station I was listening to. They might have thought I had won some big prize, and essentially I really had. This was it! My big chance was close at hand. Maybe the hypoglycemic episodes would finally end.

I kept a packed bag in the trunk of the car, ready to go at all times, just like when I was pregnant. After eating dinner, I took the Metro train to NIH so we would not have two cars on the campus, since my husband would be coming later. Also, you can never be sure about traffic conditions in the Washington, D.C. area. When I arrived at NIH, I quickly checked in with admissions. I had already completed all the paper work and registered early to avoid any delays at this point in the process. Dr. Harlan came to my room and told me that the pancreas had just arrived. There had been a fire in one of the Metro tunnels earlier, and the courier had been instructed to find an alternative way to get to NIH. Thank goodness, I had no problem with the Metro.

I waited patiently in my room for the next step, and tried to read but found that impossible. Around eleven o'clock that night, things began to happen. The radiologist, Dr. Richard Chang, came to my room and did a preliminary scan with a portable x-ray machine to locate my portal vein, the main vein that leads into the liver. It is deep within the body, so it takes some skill to locate it. Dr. Chang explained again what would happen during the transplant procedure. He told me that he would locate the portal vein and a catheter would be inserted into the vein. A catheter is a hollow flexible tube for insertion into a body cavity, duct, or vessel to allow the passage of fluids. The islets would be in a solution and they would be infused into my liver through this tube. Scientists have tried different locations for the islet infusion but most agree that the portal vein is best, and it has been used as the islet transplant location for more than 20 years. The liver has been used for many reasons. The first reason is that research has shown that the islets can function there. When insulin is normally produced by the pancreas in people who do not have diabetes, the first place it goes is to the liver via the portal vein. The liver is a main site of action for insulin. In addition, animal studies suggest that the liver represents a site that is relatively "privileged" with regard to the immune system. It may be that it is easier to prevent rejection of islet cells in the liver than in other locations.

Dr. Harlan planned to infuse the islets into my liver. He visited again and explained the risks one last time. He told me that I could choose to not go ahead with the procedure, and that it was totally up to me. It was now close to 1:30 a.m., and the team was just getting ready to take me down to the operating room. I assured him that I wanted to proceed. I was filled with anticipation from head to toe. He requested that I sign an informed consent form again, just in case I had changed my mind since the last time I had signed one. I readily complied, and he left to prepare for the procedure.

Then my nurse told me it was time to go down to the radiology suite. They put me on a gurney and we went down to the first floor from the eleventh. The building was very eerily quiet at that time of night and there was no one around. The whole place had a ghost town appearance very different from the hustling and bustling atmosphere during the day. The "delivery" person steering the gurney was a very recent employee and she was not sure exactly where to go. We ended up cruising around in circles, and stopped to ask directions from a maintenance worker, the only person around at that time of night. I began to become a little concerned that I would miss the whole thing because we were lost, and I felt a little like the man who never returned from riding the MTA beneath the streets of Boston (in the song by the Kingston Trio). After a few revolutions around the first floor, we eventually did find the right room in the radiology suite.

A large group of people were waiting for us in the suite. They had wondered what had happened to us. We realized no one was in the halls because they were all here in the room waiting for us. When we arrived, the radiologist started to locate my portal vein. After a few tries he found it, and they were ready to start the procedure. They gave me a local anesthetic and numbed the spot under my right breast where they inserted the catheter. They administered a small amount of sedative and monitored me to see if I would fall asleep. But I didn't want to miss this! I have a vague memory of Dr. Harlan standing there waiting, holding a glass syringe filled with a greenish-yellow solution. The image is vague because I had to remove my contact lenses for the procedure. I really wanted to see those islets! Dr. Harlan moved forward and slowly started to infuse the solution. I was awake and discussed how I felt throughout the whole procedure. A glucose drip and an insulin drip kept my blood sugars steady. They took my blood sugar many times throughout the procedure so they could make the proper adjustments. When the islet injection was complete after about two hours, they removed the catheter. At around 4 a.m., they took me back to my room and the whole thing was finished. Dr. Hirschberg, an endocrine fellow, was assigned to stay with me in my room to monitor how everything was progressing. They expected that some of the islets would slough off and die. As their last hurrah, those dying islets released insulin. As mine died, I had my last hypoglycemic episode. It was only a slight reaction, and they were able to adjust my glucose level quickly to compensate. I remained on my side for a few hours just to decrease the chance of bleeding from where the catheter had been inserted.

The islets immediately starting doing their job of producing insulin. The team frequently monitored my glucose levels, but not every fifteen minutes, as before.

The time between tests was slowly lengthened. For me, it was simple procedure—sure, I just lay there. Everyone else was working very hard.

A small adhesive bandage just under my right breast covered the infusion site. They had reached the portal vein through my ribs. I felt a tiny bit of discomfort at the site right after the procedure, but it was really a painless procedure. Excitement kept me going throughout the day despite my sleepless night. By midmorning I was up and calling all my relatives to tell them the good news. When I called my brother Tom, I said, "Guess where I am?" When I told him I was in the hospital he said, "Oh, no. Not again." I cheerfully went on to explain that this was a good hospital stay this time.

During that day, many people came to visit with me. The pharmacologist came and explained the medication I would be taking and their possible side effects. A chart listing all the medication, dosages, when I was scheduled to take them and possible side effects filled a sheet of paper. A nutritionist came to explain foods to be avoided and safety precautions to take with food and water since my immune system would be depressed. The only food restriction was grapefruit. Grapefruit interferes with the efficiency of the drugs I was taking. My doctors were in and out of my room all day. All of them were very caring and took a lot of time to answer all my questions. One event that really meant a lot to me was a visit by the technicians from the lab who had spent six hours preparing the islets for me the previous night. The whole team of four came to see the person who had received the cells. They wished me well, and I expressed my gratitude to them. The procedure was definitely a team effort. Everyone was very excited that things were going so well.

All told, an estimated 420,000 islets were injected into my body. That equals 7,000 islets per kilogram of weight. The Edmonton protocol typically required 10,000 islets per kilogram of weight, to be accomplished in two infusions. Dr. Harlan told me that they would monitor my progress, and decide later when (or if) the second infusion would be given. As it turns out, I have done so well that, so far, I have only required one transplant.

On Friday, they felt I was well stabilized, and my husband took me home. Since I was advised to take it easy, I refrained from exercise that weekend. On Monday, I went to work. I was still taking insulin through the pump, because Dr. Harlan wanted the islets to become comfortable in their new location. He didn't want them to be under too much stress and have to work too hard. The islets were now living in my liver but they still needed to make their permanent residence in their new home—moving the furniture around, hanging up the pictures, and meeting the neighbors. I continued to take my blood sugars eight times a day; that is, before and after each meal, at bedtime and at 3 a.m. I communicated the results to my doctors daily. I also took my weight, temperature, and blood pressure every morning. Over the next 11 days, my requirements for injected insulin decreased steadily. On June 25, 11 days after the transplant, the team told me: "Take the pump off. Let's give it a try!" I removed the pump, and the islets were on their own. They have functioned well since then!

But, that's not the end of the story.

Chapter 8
MEDICATION AND SIDE EFFECTS

Even before the transplant took place, I started taking medicine to prevent rejection of the islets. I received an intravenous injection of Daclizumab (Zenapax) immediately before I received the transplant, while the lab team was preparing the islets. Over the next two months, I returned to NIH every two weeks to receive four more injections of this drug.

Another immunosuppressive drug I take is Tacrolimus (Prograf, FK 506), in tablet form. Sirolimus (rapamune, rapamycin) is the third immunosuppressive drug that is part of the research. Previous to this time, transplant recipients received steroids to keep their bodies from rejecting their new organs. However, there was a major problem with the steroids because they appear to be toxic to islets. Tacrolimus and Sirolimus were newer drugs first used for islet transplant recipients by the team in Edmonton. The levels of these drugs are adjusted depending on lab results. Initially, I took a liquid form of Sirolimus, which I had to mix with orange juice. I now take Sirolimus in a tablet form. These medications reduce the risk of rejection by limiting T lymphocyte (also called T cell) activity. The T cells destroyed my islets cells in the first place and caused my diabetes. The major objective was to prevent my T cells from doing that again with the new islets.

One of the side effects that I suffered with Sirolimus is mouth ulcers. During the first year after transplant, I had major mouth ulcers. They completely filled the inside of my cheeks. My doctors would send me down to dentistry to have specialists provide treatment. They would check in my mouth and quickly call in all the other dentists, interns, and fellows to have a look because they were all impressed with how spectacular the ulcers were. At one point, they even brought out a huge camera with an enormous lens to take a picture of my mouth. They wanted to include them in a medical textbook. After a few visits and many pictures, I wanted them to include a picture of my face—not just the inside of my mouth. The dentist attempted to humor me, but because the lens was so large, he had to keep backing up until he was flat against the opposite wall. While I still wonder if my face will ever appear in those textbooks—I'm sure my "prize-winning" ulcers will. The dental professionals did give me a solution called chlorhexidine (Peridex), which I use as a preventive mouth rinse. This solution appears to help and has diminished the severity and frequency of the ulcers. But I continued to get ulcers for 18 months after the transplant. They typically occurred when the level of Sirolimus in my body was too high. Since my levels have been relatively steady, the occurrence of mouth ulcers has decreased. Twice a day, I take one prescription lozenge, clotrimazole (Mycelex Troches), to lessen the chance of mouth fungal infections. I occasionally continue to get fever blisters on my lips, but they are relatively minor.

During the first year after transplant I also took a low dose of co-trimoxazole (Bactrim)—a medicine that helps prevent infection from certain pathogens otherwise common in patients taking immunosuppressive drugs—three times a day as a preventive measure. Multivitamins, magnesium, calcium, and aspirin also are a part of my daily routine.

For the first few days after the procedure, I had to give myself an injection of a drug called Lovenox which is a low molecular weight heparin, to thin my blood and help prevent clotting within the portal vein where the infusion had taken place (the medical care team and I had to walk a tightrope between internal bleeding, and clotting following the transplant procedure). I had thought I was finally done with giving myself injections, but not quite yet. I only had to do that for a short time, and it was certainly worth it. I didn't experience any bleeding or clotting.

Another side effect of the drugs for me is an elevated cholesterol level. To counter that side effect, I take Simvastatin (Zocor). And I correct elevated blood pressure, another side effect, by taking lisinopril (Prinivil, Zestril).

Edema, caused by excess fluid in the body, is another side effect that has been very persistent in my ankles. Others have noted it in their hands and face as well. This problem is, of course, made worse by flying. I returned from an eight-hour flight from Hungary with really huge, puff pastry-like ankles. I called NIH and the doctors advised me to elevate my feet. I thought that if some elevation was good then a lot of elevation would be better, so I accomplished this by standing on my head, against a wall, using two chairs as props. This really did the trick, and my ankles returned to normal size after a few minutes of being upside down. A few hours after applying what I thought was a very effective technique, a person in my office asked what was wrong with my face, and told me I had a rash. I rushed to look in the mirror and saw that there were two very large red blotches on my face near my temples. I called NIH and they made an immediate appointment for me in dermatology. A rash is a common side effect of the drugs I am taking. I stopped by to see my doctors on the way to dermatology and they confirmed that I did indeed have red blotches on my face. Up in dermatology, Dr. Maria Turner started asking me questions. She didn't think the marks looked like a rash, but she was not yet sure what was going on. She asked if I had eaten anything unusual, and other questions along that line. When she asked about my recent activities and heard I had been standing on my head, she rolled her eyes and said, "Of course!" She told me I had broken some blood vessels. Dr. Harlan and the NIH team said that they'll have to change the protocol for islet transplant recipients to prohibit headstands. I wonder how many people this will discourage from applying.

Because my immune system is suppressed so it will not destroy my new islets, I have a much harder time fighting infections. Before my transplant, my doctors told me that I would not necessarily get more infections, but that they would tend to escalate into severe infections quickly. In the fall shortly after transplant, I was working in the garden turning the earth for the next season. A few days later I noticed a red spot on my left hand. It grew bigger over the next few days. I called NIH and the doctors wanted to see me right away. A referral to dermatology got me in to see Dr. Turner again. She looked at the spot carefully and said she was uncertain whether it was a bacterial or fungal infection. She took a biopsy, which was the only way to get a definite identification. The biopsy was inconclusive, so she took another one a few days later. The second one also was inconclusive and they were still not able to determine the nature of the infection. I went back for a third biopsy. They had to diagnose it before treatment could begin, because if they prescribed fungal medication, those drugs would affect the immunosuppressive drugs, and they would have to monitor my drug levels very closely. If the infection was bacterial, the treatment would be a general antibiotic and there would be no interactions with the other drugs. Because they were having difficulty determining the exact nature of the infection, they invited me to participate in "grand rounds." This meant that about 100 dermatologists, internists, and fellows came in over the course of an hour to look at my hand. It became routine for me. When a group would enter the room, I simply held out my hand. One of the doctors commented that I presented very well. The doctors discussed my case in a symposium, and finally determined that the infection was fungal. I started treatment immediately and the infection cleared up quickly. I had to have my blood levels checked frequently and my drug levels were adjusted accordingly throughout the treatment.

I got another major infection while hiking in Yosemite National Park in the summer of 2002. A group of friends, relatives, and my husband and I went to California for a week of glorious hiking and partying. I wore some old hiking boots until one day I found myself slipping on a difficult trail. My sister, Ann, graciously traded boots with me since hers had a little more tread than mine. We both noticed that evening that we had a little rash on our legs. Her rash cleared up by the next day. Mine was red, hot, swelling, and spreading. Throughout that day it continued to swell and spread, but I kept hiking, albeit a little slower. By the end of that day the rash was quite inflamed. One of the members of our group was a doctor, so I consulted him. He advised me to elevate my leg and put ice on it, which I did. There is a small clinic in Yosemite, and my husband dragged me over there. By this time, all my little cuts and scrapes had become inflamed. They immediately determined that I had a systemic bacterial infection. Of course, they had never treated anyone who had received an islet cell transplant, so I was quite the celebrity. After consulting with an NIH doctor, they gave me a general antibiotic shot, and an oral antibiotic. The infection began to subside by the next day. I did refrain from hiking, and kept my leg elevated and iced for the entire day. By the next day, I was back up and walking again.

I had another experience with infection when I noticed some fungal growth under one fingernail and three toe nails. Fortunately my doctors treated this with a topical solution that is slowly clearing up the fungal growth after a year.

In the spring of 2003, I was cleaning up a patch of English Ivy and other plants in a corner of the front yard. I do this at the beginning of every season, but this year, I had an adverse reaction to the plants. Neither I nor my husband could see any obvious poison ivy, but my body reacted to some kind of irritation. Many areas of my skin were inflamed and blistering. After yet another trip to NIH and another consultation with dermatology, they gave me a prescription cream that stopped the itching.

In the fall of 2003 I was exposed to a child with a cough. Another child present developed a cough and a fever, but recovered in a few days. Over the same few days, my symptoms progressed from a slight cough to pneumonia. During the worst part, I experienced five days of intense illness. Then, it cleared up over the next few weeks. Once again, strong antibiotics helped me to recover.

While the above list of side effects is already a long one, there were still more to come. In my first year I experienced some gastrointestinal problems with diarrhea. Fortunately, during the second year these episodes occurred less and less frequently. They did require some quick trips to the bathroom, but they were never major and usually lasted for only a few hours.

Five months after transplant, the doctors were not satisfied with my blood sugar levels. They felt they were running too high. A potential danger with high blood sugars is that they can damage islets by making them work too hard. It is essential that the vitality of islets be maintained so they prescribed metformin (Glucophage, Glucophage XR) to decrease the amount of sugar my liver produced, which appeared to do the trick. In the summer of 2003, they also added pioglitazone (Actos) to improve my sensitivity to insulin. However, this did not appear to be sufficient because my fasting blood sugars continued to creep up, approaching the pre-diabetic range. A small dose of Lantus insulin (3 units) was prescribed in early October 2003, twenty-eight months after transplant. My fasting blood sugars then returned to an acceptable range below 110. The decision to take insulin was not an easy one for me. I was extremely frightened that the hypoglycemic reactions would return. Dr. Harlan assured me that he did not think this would happen since the dose was so low. He felt, however, that it would be sufficient to protect the islets. Since I am an important member of my treatment team they respected my thoughts on the subject and waited until I was willing to give it a try. I did consent due to the risk to the islets. I have experienced no reactions since starting the low dose.

Another very common side effect of the immunosuppressive drugs is fatigue. Luckily, I haven't experienced that side effect. I have always been a very active person with lots of energy, and that has not changed. I still take a dance aerobics class twice a week. In the winter, my husband and I enjoy skiing, both downhill and cross country. In the other seasons we bike, frequently covering distances of thirty to forty miles, and also hike. I walk for at least thirty minutes almost every day. I enjoy ice-skating, swimming, and horseback riding.

Even though I have experienced many side effects—and all of them are distracting, disgusting, and/or painful—they have been minor inconveniences compared to the alternatives. These included the possibility of permanent brain damage, or death from extreme hypoglycemia (or injury to others, for example, in a car accident). No matter how bad it gets, it's better for me than the alternatives. With the proper medicine, my infections have cleared up and I have been able to tolerate all the other side effects, so far.

These side effects and others have occurred in other transplant patients to various degrees. For some, they were debilitating and incapacitating. Diarrhea and fatigue prevented some from even leaving their homes. Their bodies just couldn't tolerate the drugs. Some contracted infections that did not respond to treatment with medication. Some had to stop taking their immunosuppressive drugs to enable antibiotics to work. Their bodies then rejected the transplanted islets.

Although the transplants may have been successful for some, and the immediate effects may have been highly beneficial, the frequent occurrence of severe side effects led Dr. Harlan and the NIH team to become greatly concerned. They have truly considered the trade-offs and weighed the advantages and disadvantages of doing the islet transplants versus continuing with diabetes management. Now, they question the wisdom of trading one drug (insulin) for others (Sirolimus and Prograf).

Researchers have proven that it is possible to isolate and transplant islet cells from a donor pancreas into a person with Type 1 diabetes. They have successfully done this over 300 times world-wide, as of this writing. Research emphasis is now on developing new drugs to prevent rejection, and on eliminating the need for immunosuppressive drugs all together. This problem has not yet been solved.

Chapter 9
HEART PANIC

About one week after the transplant, the doctors told me I could start exercising again and engage in more strenuous activity. They felt pretty certain that my islets were comfortable in their new home. Every day at work I enjoyed walking during lunchtime with various office mates. However, they were not always enthusiastic about going along, either because of the weather, which did include rain and snow, or because of not having the right shoes. One day I was able to convince my friend Sue to join me. We started out quickly and a stab of pain in my chest slowed me right down. After we slowed down, the pain went away and we continued walking. After we returned to the office, I checked with my NIH team, and they advised me to call my HMO to have things checked out. At an urgent care appointment that evening, the doctors took an EKG and told me all was well. The cardiologist on duty suggested I take a stress test at his office the next day. When I called the office the next morning, they immediately set up an appointment for me that afternoon. After a long wait at the office, they finally "squeezed" me in, and started the test. Once again, I felt like the bionic woman with the heart monitor and leads hooked up. When I started running on the treadmill, it took quite a while for my heart rate to reach the desired level. Throughout the test, I spoke with the nurse, who was very interested in the details of my islet cell transplant and the procedure.

After the stress test, the nurse congratulated me on what good shape I was in. She said she would share the results with the cardiologist and that he would get back to me. He called the next day and told me the results were within normal limits, but that he wanted me to take some medication as a precautionary measure. I took a beta blocker for about two weeks. He also gave me some nitroglycerine to carry with me should I experience any sharp pains again, which I didn't. We decided to discontinue the medication. The cardiologist felt my quick start that day had caused the pain.

A few days after the stress test, I received a very warm and friendly personal note from the nurse who had administered the stress test. She told me she really admired me for what I had done and that she considered me a pioneer. I really appreciated her taking the time to write me a personnel note. I had never thought of myself in those terms. Desperate to stop my escalating hypoglycemic episodes, I signed up for the experimental procedure hoping for a solution. I am hopeful that the data the NIH team is collecting will help in the continued search for a cure that will benefit all who endure diabetes.

Chapter 10
SIROLIMUS STRESS

On August 9, 2001, almost two months after the transplant, Pete and I traveled to Hungary for a big Berty family reunion, from August 20th to the 26th. We flew over early so we could visit Slovakia and hike in the High Tatra Mountains as we had done once before. We were scheduled to return home on August 27. When we purchased our tickets, I also bought some traveler's insurance so that if I needed a second transplant, and a donor pancreas become available, I would be able to fly back immediately.

When I discussed the details of our plans with the team at NIH, they agreed that we could work it out. They wanted my blood drawn weekly and sent back to NIH. They gave me my last infusion of the immunosuppressive drug Daclizumab the day before we left. They also gave me all the supplies I would need to have my blood drawn while out of the county, including tubes, needles, alcohol wipes, and FedEx boxes. They needed to monitor my immunosuppressive drug levels so appropriate adjustments could be made if necessary. We sent many e-mail messages to our relatives in Hungary explaining what would be needed. Planning things in advance, we thought, might make the process easier. This was not an easy task either for us or for our family in Hungary. But they assured us that all requests were within the realm of possibility. We knew that we could communicate with the team at NIH, so we were set to go.

On the eve of our departure, I counted the number of each drug that I would need for the time we would be gone. I was taking approximately ten different medications and vitamins at this time. I also had to account for the different scheduling for each drug each day. Some of the drugs I counted out into a daily dosage container that holds one week's worth of medications. The others I put into ten separate containers with a label so that I could then refill the daily dosage container as we progressed on our journey. To cover any unforeseen circumstances, I threw in a little extra of each and put all those extra pills in a separate container. This whole process took more than an hour. All of the containers took up about as much space as 10 coffee mugs. They varied in size and shape. When I checked all my containers against my written list, at last I felt secure that everything was packed and ready to go.

We began our journey in Budapest and stayed until Monday, August 13th. I had blood drawn that morning and sent it via FedEx back to NIH. We took the tram to the hospital and arrived shortly after 8:00 a.m. A friend of my husband's cousin, Gábor, who was a doctor at the hospital, had agreed to help us, and he set up the appointment. Even though the doctor was not at the hospital, his nurses were expecting us. We quickly located them and started the process. It was not easy, however, to communicate that we only needed the blood drawn and centrifuged. They didn't understand why no lab work was required. Of course, my husband was doing all the talking in his native Hungarian. The hospital personnel were not interested in using any of the equipment I had brought with me. Instead, they pulled out one huge tube and one very large needle to draw my blood. After a few unsuccessful attempts, the nurse decided to call in an "expert." This was a very familiar situation for me, since this had happened many times in the past. The expert was more successful, and managed in only three tries. She then used the big tube of blood to fill all my little tubes. We took the tubes down to the laboratory and the technicians placed them in their centrifuge machine. While we waited for that to be finished, Pete left to find the rental car delivery agents who were supposed to meet us at one of the hospital entrances. After several phone calls and trips in and out of the hospital, he finally found them. We drove to the FedEx office, and mailed the blood without too much hassle.

We arrived in Stary Smokovec, Slovakia, on Tuesday and checked into a small bed and breakfast. We hiked for eight hours the next day; six hours to get up the mountain and only two hours to get down. It was a rather steep hike. Having discovered that we could use the Internet at our B&B only after 9 p.m., we tried that night and had to wait for other people to finish. Using the Internet, we also could check e-mail messages sent to our home e-mail address, which is how we received messages. The service was poor, and we often lost the connection. Eventually we were able to read an e-mail message from NIH. They had received the blood sample, analyzed it, and recommended an increase in the amount of Sirolimus I was taking. This was important, since it was one of the immunosuppressive drugs I was taking to prevent rejection of my new islets.

That evening, when I took out all my pill bottles I had spent hours counting out, I put the pills in my container that held a week's worth of drugs, reflecting the recommended increase. Counting out my Sirolimus supply, I realized I didn't have enough in that bottle. Thinking I would use the extra pills, I searched for the big bottle containing Sirolimus. Looking in my shoulder bag, I couldn't find them. I dumped everything out of that bag and my suitcase and purse, searching frantically to find the rest of my supply. I couldn't find it! I didn't have it! How could this happen? Panic was beginning to set in. What could I possibly do from here in Slovakia? I had enough pills to get me through Monday with a half dose of Sirolimus for Tuesday, but no more. Hurrying back downstairs, I sent another e-mail message with the "URGENT-NEED MEDS" in the subject line. It was quite late by that time and I tried to go to sleep, but didn't have much luck.

I had to wait until 9 p.m. the next day to get a response from NIH. We had planned a hike again that day, and when we realized there was nothing we could do at that point we went ahead with the original plan. We had talked for many hours about our options. We planned to return to Hungary the next day. Since we had many contacts there, we were hopeful they would be able to help us.

That day, my husband and I started out together and after a few hours he went on ahead and hiked to the summit. Traveling at a much slower pace, I turned around earlier. That gave me some time to do some solitary thinking. With a sense of impending doom, I tried to explore all my options, and attempted to come up with a plan of action. If I did not get the drug, I knew I would have to return to the United States a week ahead of plan. I was certainly not willing to take a chance that my body would reject the islets.

Arriving back in town at the bottom of the hill, I ventured into a small shop. Using all of my limited Hungarian skills (many in Slovakia speak Hungarian), I was able ask if there was an Internet café in town, and for directions there. Another customer responded to me, in English, that she knew where the café was and that

94

she was going to pass by there herself. She offered to take me there. So much for my Hungarian skills!

While walking over to the café, we introduced ourselves. She told me she had a respiratory condition and that she was in this mountain town to recover. I told her of my transplant and my current dilemma. Much to my surprise, she told me she was a plastic surgeon from the Czech Republic. She offered to go to the pharmacy with me to try to locate the medication. She spoke to the pharmacist, who informed us that she did not have the drug but that she would get online and check in another, bigger town to see if they might possibly have a supply. Unfortunately, they did not.

The Internet café was close by. We went there and found it was simply a corner of a restaurant with two computers. Customers paid by the minute and the rate was very inexpensive. People were using both computers and others were waiting to use them. Because of the six hour time difference, I realized it was still too early for anyone to be at NIH yet, and decided to return later.

That evening we again tried to send e-mail from our B&B. Once again, we were not successful and kept losing the connection. We spoke to the son of the owners of the B&B, who had been helping us using his limited English, and begged him for permission to place a telephone call. We offered to pay, and he graciously agreed. I called NIH and spoke with Lisa, my transplant coordinator. She was a little anxious for me, but offered some hope of a solution. She would ship the drug via FedEx to me. That was a relief. We hung up, and I felt certain it would be on the way and my worries would be over. Little did we know what lay ahead.

We called our relatives in Hungary and told them to expect a package for me on Friday—no problem. We traveled back to Hungary and arrived early Friday evening, but the package had not arrived! We were staying in Veszprém, a small university town about an hour and a half from Budapest, and close to Lake Balaton. We were staying with my husband's cousin, András, his wife, Teodóra, and their family. At their home, Internet access was not limited by the same restrictions we had faced in Slovakia. They had a good internet provider and we were able to get online quickly. I sent an e-mail message to try to get the tracking number for the FedEx package. Because of customs regulations regarding the shipping of drugs, FedEx would not be able to deliver them until Thursday, which was too late. Dr. Harlan did send me an e-mail message and told me that the half-life of Sirolimus was 24 hours, and so I could make it until Tuesday with a half dose that morning.

With the new information about the half-life of the drug I felt a little relief. But that still might not be good enough, I thought, because FedEx could not deliver until Thursday. We discussed this for a while, and came up with a backup plan. Pete's parents were flying to Budapest and would arrive on Wednesday. We hoped the team at NIH could get the drug to them in Allentown, Pennsylvania, and that they could carry it with them. The timing was close, since they would be leaving their home the next morning to go the airport in New York. I called Lisa and explored this possibility with her. She said they would certainly try. We called Pete's parents to tell them about the plan. The NIH team used FedEx to send an overnight express package to them in Allentown. We waited anxiously for the phone call telling us the package had arrived. That call finally did come, and I knew the drugs would arrive by late in the day Wednesday. This was still very risky. There was still a high likelihood that things might go wrong. The real possibility still existed that my body would reject the islets. I was still anxious to get the Sirolimus on Tuesday at the latest.

I decided to alert my traveler's insurance company that I might need to fly home on Tuesday. A representative told me that another service they provided was tracking down medications for people who were traveling. That was exciting news. They started their search. After numerous phone calls, they discovered that my medication was not available in England, but that it may be in Vienna, Austria (which would be a day trip). Teo, in whose home we were staying and causing all this havoc, is a very gifted linguist. She speaks Hungarian, German, and English. She called the hospital where we had been told the drug was located. After many transfers, she determined that they didn't have the medication. The insurance representatives once again assured me it was there, and that they would follow up. They called back a few hours later and gave me the name of the doctor we should speak with. Teo called again and learned that Frau Doctor would be there on Sunday between 12 p.m. and 3 p.m. So for now on Saturday, that road was closed.

Meanwhile, Teo called the transplant hospitals in Hungary to see if they knew of the drug and where we might find it. Staff members at one of the hospitals told her that at one time they did have some, but that it was no longer available. Still no luck.

After a search on the Internet, we found the formula for the drug. Teo, Pete, and I went to the local pharmacy with the formula and asked if they had the medicine or if they could make it. Teo pleaded my case to no avail. They couldn't help us.

Back at NIH, Lisa and the pharmacist were trying to solve the problem. It was now Saturday, and they were frantically trying to find a way to get the drug to me. They contacted the manufacturer to see where it might be available in Europe. They told her that they couldn't locate it anywhere in Europe. They then switched back to pursuing how to ship the drug to me. They contacted a shipping company and explained the situation to an associate there named Patrick. He assured them his company could get it to me. Lisa rushed over to the shipping company and hand delivered the drug to them. They shipped it out that day, and we were told that it would arrive on Monday. Little did they know that Monday was to be a huge national holiday, the culmination of a year's celebration of the millennial anniversary of the birth of Hungary. Via e-mail messages and phone calls, I gave Patrick the news and he assured me that I would get the drug on Tuesday.

On Tuesday morning, Teo started calling the local office of the shipping company in Budapest at 8 a.m. A sleepy voice told her to wait a little while because it was the day after the holiday, and that we should call back in an hour after everyone got up and moving. We waited an hour and Teo called again. This time, she was told that the shipment had arrived but that they had to get it through customs. He also told her that we had to get some documents to them so that they could do that. He asked if we could do that in the next couple of days. Days? We didn't have the luxury of taking our time. Teo told him that she would immediately fax the documents to him, and once again explained the immediacy of the situation. She manages a small customs office and is very familiar with customs regulations, so she faxed the papers to him along with the section of the customs laws concerning life-threatening situations. Well, it really wasn't life threatening, but my NIH team might have considered threatening my life at that point.

Teo returned home around 11:00 a.m. after sending all the papers and a strongly worded message. Apparently, the company usually waited until they filled a truck before they delivered all the goods that had been shipped. In my case, NIH had arranged for immediate shipment just so there would be no such delays, and the company said they would send it right out. Patrick was instrumental in the process. So, the wait began. Throughout the day, many people came and went from the house. Each time the doorbell rang, we all jumped up to see who was there. That happened many times. By the end of the day, there was quite a gathering of relatives and friends at the house. Finally, at 4 p.m. the doorbell rang and 12 people jumped up and ran to the door. It was the delivery person with the precious package! Everyone clapped and cheered, but no one was louder than me. The overwhelmed delivery person sheepishly looked around wide eyed and gingerly handed over the package, I ripped it open and took out the pills with tears of gratitude in my eyes.

Chapter 11
WHAT A DIFFERENCE!

Five days after the transplant, I attended a big dinner that was a very loud affair, and I was telling a friend about my recent islet transplant. Her eyes widened, and she moved a little closer to me, with her mouth agape. She regained her composure and asked, "Who is your plastic surgeon?" I stared back at her speechless and with a very quizzical look on my face. I told her again that I had an islet transplant. She burst out laughing and said, "Oh my goodness, I thought you said eyelid transplant!"

The difference the transplant has made in my life and to my family and friends is almost indescribable. I can eat now when I am hungry. This is a new phenomenon for me. I have lost almost 15 pounds since the transplant because I no longer have to eat all the time to cover all my low blood sugars. My friends and family are relieved, to say the least. They no longer have to keep on eye on me to see if I have "The Look," or if I'm sweating. I can actually skip a meal if I choose to. My husband asks, "Why would you ever want to skip a meal?" And I respond, "Just because I can!" But I still think like I have diabetes. A 40-year habit is hard to break. While stuck in traffic my first thoughts are, "How long will this last? Will I have enough food to cover a low if I'm stuck here for a long time?" Then I catch myself, smack my forehead, and say, "Wait, I don't have to do that anymore!"

Also, I no longer experience the enormous range of glucose levels, from lows of 0 to highs of more than 400. To say the least, this change has evened out my life. I haven't had any hypoglycemic episodes since the day of the transplant, and one of my lowest readings was an 85 after a 90-minute run. The highest blood sugar I have experienced post transplant has been about 170 two hours after eating. I can ride my bike 40 miles and still have a blood sugar of 114 when I'm finished. In the past, after exercise, my blood sugar would drop for hours, sometimes throughout the night. The transplant has certainly changed my perspective of highs and lows, and my blood sugars are within a much narrower range. I am enjoying much better blood sugar control.

The A1c is a test that measures a person's average blood glucose level over the previous 2 to 3 months. My A1c level before transplant was 8.8, which is relatively high. The normal level for a person without diabetes is below 6.4. Since transplant they have ranged from 5.8 to 6.4. But the most important benefit of all is that I no longer have any hypoglycemic episodes and therefore certainly no hypoglycemia unawareness.

Shortly after the transplant, I was able to answer phones at our hospital during the terrorist crisis for many hours without having to worry about food or blood sugars. I was in such a rush when I left my home, I didn't even take my meter with me. I didn't eat breakfast either, and I ate a doughnut after I arrived at the hospital.

I continue to measure my temperature, weight, and blood pressure daily. I now only take my blood sugars twice a day, rather than eight to twelve times a day as I did before my transplant when I was experiencing hypoglycemic reactions. I was also taking my blood sugar every time I got in the car to drive. My fingertips certainly appreciate that relief. I send all this information to the team at NIH on a biweekly basis. Every month I go to NIH to have lab work done. Once every three months, they conduct an arginine test. My time commitment to the clinical trial has decreased significantly since the initial transplant. Initially, I was having lab work done weekly and an arginine test done monthly. Of course, if anything arises at any time that I or the team feels concerned about, I see a specialist immediately. If the doctors change my medications, then a follow up blood draw is needed to assess the effect of the change. I am very well known at the Clinical Center at NIH and all the people there are part of my team. Every time I go, I stay for a long time because I stop in so many different departments to let everyone know how I'm doing. They are all as thrilled as I am with my success.

In September 2001, three months after transplant, I was once again signing up for my aerobics class and came to the part concerning health conditions. I was so excited when I marked a great big "NO" next to the question about diabetes.

Pete now says that diabetes is not a pervasive presence in our lives. Not everything we do has to revolve around my eating, exercise, and insulin schedule. In addition, he is relieved that the police are not calling him at all hours of the day and night. He says that he can now sleep through the whole night without keeping a part of his brain alert for any signs of a reaction.

Once, my sister Paula was at a doctor's appointment and the doctor took a family history. My sister proudly said, "My sister used to have diabetes." "Type 1?" the doctor incredulously asked. My sister's positive response prompted a whole series of questions, and she got to tell my story.

Back in my office, an ambulance raced by our windows with lights flashing and sirens screaming. My friend Joyce, who had come to my rescue many times in the past, jumped up and shouted, "Not here! Not for Ellen anymore!"

A major change for me is that I have regained my independence. I felt I was becoming a burden to my husband, family, and friends when the rate and intensity of my hypoglycemia episodes increased. Out of their concern for me, they found it necessary to keep a close watch on my behavior. I would not have survived without my support network. My reactions always interrupted activities. My family and friends would sigh with resignation as they would have to stop what they were doing and attend to my condition, yet again. The transplant has brought tremendous relief for them, but also for me. Gaining back my confidence in my ability to take care of myself, I have much more control over the variables in my life. I am not at the mercy of a million different factors that could cause me to lose consciousness at any time. I don't have to worry continually or be diligent about those things. Because more of the variables are now within my control, I have more freedom to be spontaneous. Life is not so perilous and regimented, and I now drive with much more confidence. I no longer have to depend on others to bring me back to reality after falling over the crumbling edge of the hypoglycemic cliff.

I am thrilled with the results of the transplant in my case. It has been a success, and I have not suffered major side effects from the drugs. But that is not true for all transplant recipients. Research needs to continue before this becomes a viable option for all those with diabetes. And, there is a major problem with the limited supply of islets available for transplant. There are simply not enough organ donors—and even if islets were harvested from every organ donor, there still wouldn't be enough to go around. Other sources of islets need to be investigated. Another major drawback to the procedure is the side effects of the immunosuppressive drugs. When those two major hurdles are overcome, I have great hope that this will lead to the cure. The long-term results are not available yet. The procedure is still too new.

I am grateful that my glucometer is a fast read, so I only have to hold my breath for five seconds before seeing my blood sugar reading. And I do hold my breath—every time—as I wait to see if my islets are still working. And so far, they are. I am very grateful to my NIH team for the outstanding care I have received. Doctors David Harlan and Boaz Hirshberg have been on both the treatment and follow-up team. Doctors Kristina Rother and Benigno Digon have joined my follow-up team and Trish Koussis is now my nurse coordinator.

My ultimate fantasy is that a person with Type 1 diabetes will be able to visit their doctor's office, be diagnosed, receive new islet cells, and be cured—all in a single visit.

But for now, after 40 years and 22,000 shots of insulin, I can shout from the rooftops, "I used to have Type 1 diabetes!"

Chapter 12
EPILOG

Since my transplant, I have spoken to many organizations and groups about my experience. I have spoken at the national meetings of both the Juvenile Diabetes Research Foundation and the American Diabetes Association and at local meetings of the same groups around the country. The Diabetes Wellness Foundation and Diabetes Educators also have invited me to speak. In addition, I have spoken at local support groups, and to many individuals about my experience.

The response I get from every talk is overwhelming. Many parents whose children have diabetes tell me that they just want to tell their children they have actually met someone who has been cured of Type 1 diabetes. They often tell me that it is thrill to meet a real person who has been cured, instead of just reading about the statistical results of experiments.

While traveling on a speaking engagement in Hawaii, I met a man who had been diagnosed with diabetes in 1938. He told me he was very grateful he had actually seen the day when someone was finally cured. He said he had been waiting sixty-four years for that to happen.

In every group that I address, there are people who have a great passion to find a cure for diabetes. Many have been working tirelessly to raise funds so research can continue. They often want to have their pictures taken with me for use in their fundraising efforts. They can point to me and say, "See, we are making progress. Ellen is proof!" By telling my story, I hope to let people know that we are moving closer to a cure. They often tell me that I have given them new inspiration to continue.

The first time I was ever asked for my autograph was in Hawaii, after I had been featured in a newspaper article and had been interviewed on a morning television talk show. A man asked for my autograph to prove to people that he was actually there, and that I was a reality. I was so overwhelmed that I almost forgot how to spell my name. He also asked my husband for his autograph as the main member of my support team.

When I speak, I am most frequently asked these questions about my experiences:

1. Do you still take your blood sugar?

Yes, twice a day—a fasting one in the morning, and then two hours after any meal. I'm still part of the clinical trial at NIH, and they need the data. I think that I would check my blood sugar anyway, even without that the NIH requirement, just to have proof that the islets are still working. The researchers can't predict how long the islets will continue to do their job, but I am counting on forever.

2. How can I get a transplant?

Details about the islet trials that are taking place in many locations around the world are available on these Web sites: Juvenile Diabetes Research Foundation (www.jdrf.org), Diabetes Station (www.diabetesstation.com), the American Diabetes Association (www.diabetes.org), and Diabetes Portal (www.diabetesport al.com). Information about clinical trials being conducted on islet transplants and many other topics is also available at www.clinicaltrials.gov.

3. Why aren't they doing islet transplants on children?

The technique is still in clinical trials, meaning it has not been done on enough people to prove that it will work. Also, it has not been in practice long enough to prove that it may be safe for children. Continued experimentation with adults hopefully will lead to safer immunosuppressive medications for children. Exploring alternative sources for islets will also assure that a supply of islets will be available. The long-term effects of the very strong immunosuppressive drugs are unknown. Can you imagine the a scenario in which a child suffers permanent and debilitating side effects of the drugs, and then a few years later, a safe cure is developed? In general, the unknowns and potential dangers to children seem to outweigh the potential benefits at this time. The hope is that safer and more effective techniques will be developed over time, and that eventually they will be made available for children.

4. What made you decide to do it?

My experiences with hypoglycemia unawareness—and their scary consequences—were what made me decide to participate in this clinical trial.

Without that complication, I probably would not have pursued it. I would have waited until that they had worked out some of the initial difficulties that they are still investigating now. My diabetes had been managed fairly well until I started to experience the hypoglycemia unawareness. However, all my efforts to avoid that complication were proving to be unsuccessful. Frequently, I was in great danger. Nothing else seemed to be available for me.

5. Would you recommend it for me?

If you aren't experiencing hypoglycemia unawareness, then I wouldn't recommend it for you. There are unknowns regarding how each individual will tolerate the drugs. There is also the danger of serious infections and difficulty clearing them up. Once researchers work out those difficulties, then the procedure will become more widely available and won't be considered experimental anymore. Until that point, my best advice is to remain in as much in control as possible, so that when the process is available, you'll be ready.

6. Would you do it again?

Yes, I would do it again without a moment's hesitation because it has eliminated my hypoglycemia. I know now how my body will tolerate the drugs, and I know what the side effects are. The transplant was a very simple, non-surgical procedure. The time commitment for collecting data, communicating with the NIH team, and going to NIH for lab work has been substantial but manageable for me.

GLOSSARY

Adapted from the NIDDK (National Institute of Digestive and Diabetes and Kidney Disease) diabetes dictionary.

A

A1c

A test that measures a person's average blood glucose level over the previous 2 to 3 months. Hemoglobin is the part of a red blood cell that carries oxygen to the body and sometimes joins with the glucose in the bloodstream. Also called hemoglobin A1c or glycosylated hemoglobin, the test shows the amount of glucose that sticks to the red blood cell, which is proportional to the amount of glucose in the blood over the life of each red blood cell. (Also called Hgb A1c.)

ACE inhibitor

An oral medicine that lowers blood pressure; ACE stands for angiotensin converting enzyme. For people with diabetes, especially those who have protein (albumin) in the urine, it also helps slow down kidney damage.

Actos

See pioglitazone.

acute

Describes something that happens suddenly and for a short time. Opposite of chronic.

adult-onset diabetes

Former term for Type 2 diabetes. Caused by the body being resistant to insulin's effect. It is no longer called adult onset because now many children diagnosed with diabetes have the disease. (The body's resistance to insulin perhaps reflects our society's increasing problems with obesity and inactivity.) In addition, some people who develop diabetes as adults actually have Type 1 diabetes because their immune systems have destroyed their beta cells. (Type 1 diabetes formerly was called juvenile onset diabetes.)

albuminuria

Condition in which the urine has more than normal amounts of a protein called albumin. Albuminuria may be a sign of nephropathy (kidney disease).

alpha cell

A type of cell in the pancreas. Alpha cells make and release a hormone called glucagon. The body sends a signal to the alpha cells to make glucagon when blood glucose falls too low. Then glucagon reaches the liver where it tells it to release glucose into the blood for energy.

antibodies

Proteins made by the body to protect itself from "foreign" substances such as bacteria or viruses. People who get Type 1 diabetes make antibodies directed against the body's own insulin-making beta cells.

Arteriosclerosis

Hardening of the arteries.

artery

A large blood vessel that carries blood with oxygen from the heart to all parts of the body.

atherosclerosis

Clogging, narrowing, and hardening of the body's large arteries and medium-sized blood vessels. Atherosclerosis can lead to stroke, heart attack, eye problems, and kidney problems.

autoimmune disease

Disorder of the body's immune system in which the immune system mistakenly attacks and destroys body tissue and thereby causes disease.

autonomic neuropathy

A type of neuropathy (nerve damage) affecting the lungs, heart, stomach, intestines, bladder, or genitals.

B

background retinopathy

A type of damage to the retina of the eye marked by bleeding, fluid accumulation, and abnormal dilation of the blood vessels. Background retinopathy is an early stage of diabetic retinopathy. Also called simple or nonproliferative retinopathy.

basal rate

A steady trickle of insulin, such as that used in insulin pumps.

beta cell

A cell that makes insulin. Beta cells are located in the islets of the pancreas.

biguanide

A class of oral medicine used to treat Type 2 diabetes that lowers blood glucose by reducing the amount of glucose produced by the liver and by helping the body respond better to insulin. (Generic name: metformin.)

blood glucose

The main sugar found in the blood and the body's main source of energy. Also called blood sugar.

blood glucose level

The amount of glucose in a given amount of blood. It is noted in milligrams per deciliter, or mg/dL.

blood glucose meter

Small, portable, battery-operated devices to test for glucose. With a typical glucose meter, the user places a small sample of blood on a disposable "test strip" and inserts the strip in the meter. The test strips are coated with chemicals (glucose oxidase, dehydrogenase, or hexokinase) that combine with glucose in blood. The meter measures how much glucose is present. Meters do this in different ways. Some measure the amount of electricity that can pass through the sample. Others measure how much light reflects from it. The meter displays the glucose level as a number. Several new models can record and store a number of test results. Some models can connect to personal computers to store or print test results.

blood glucose monitoring

Checking blood glucose level on a regular basis in order to manage diabetes.

blood pressure

The force of blood exerted on the inside walls of blood vessels. Blood pressure is expressed as a ratio (example: 120/80, read as "120 over 80"). The first number is the systolic pressure, or the pressure when the heart pushes blood out into the arteries. The second number is the diastolic pressure, or the pressure when the heart rests.

blood vessels

Tubes that carry blood to and from all parts of the body. The three main types of blood vessels are arteries, veins, and capillaries.

body mass index (bmi)

A measure of body fat based on height and weight that applies to both adult men and women. BMI is the ratio of body mass, in kilograms, to height, in meters, squared (kg/m^2). BMI is used as a guide to categorize individuals as underweight, normal weight, overweight, or obese.

BMI categories:
- Underweight: less than 18.5
- normal weight: 18.5 to 24.9
- overweight: 25 to 29.9
- obesity: 30 or greater

bolus

An extra amount of insulin taken to cover an expected rise in blood glucose, often related to a meal or snack.

borderline diabetes

A former term for impaired glucose tolerance.

brittle diabetes

A term used when a person's blood glucose level moves often from low to high and from high to low.

C

C-peptide

"Connecting peptide," a substance the pancreas releases into the bloodstream in equal amounts to insulin. A test of C-peptide levels shows how much insulin the body is making.

calorie

A unit representing the energy provided by food. Carbohydrate, protein, fat, and alcohol provide calories in the diet. Carbohydrate and protein have 4 calories per gram, fat has 9 calories per gram, and alcohol has 7 calories per gram.

capillary

The smallest of the body's blood vessels. Oxygen and glucose pass through capillary walls and enter the cells. Waste products such as carbon dioxide pass back from the cells into the blood through capillaries.

carbohydrate

One of the three main nutrients in food. Foods that provide carbohydrate are starches, vegetables, fruits, dairy products, and sugars.

carbohydrate counting

A method of meal planning for people with diabetes based on counting the number of grams of carbohydrate in food.

cardiologist

A doctor who treats people who have heart problems.

cardiovascular disease

Disease of the heart and blood vessels (arteries, veins, and capillaries).

cataract

Clouding of the lens of the eye.

catheter

A hollow flexible tube for insertion into a body cavity, duct, or vessel to allow the passage of fluids or to distend a passageway.

Chlorhexidine

A dental antibacterial, is used to prevent and treat mouth ulcers and gingivitis. Also known as Peridex.

cholesterol

A type of fat produced by the liver and found in the blood; it is also found in some foods. Cholesterol is used by the body to make hormones and build cell walls.

chronic

Describes something that is long-lasting. Opposite of acute.

circulation

The flow of blood through the body's blood vessels and heart.

Clotrimazole

An antifungal, oral medication in lozenge form, dissolved slowly in the mouth to prevent and treat mouth ulcers, also known as Mycelex Troches.

coma

A sleep-like state in which a person is not conscious. May be caused by hyperglycemia (high blood glucose) or hypoglycemia (low blood glucose) in people with diabetes.

combination therapy

The use of different medicines together (oral hypoglycemic agents or an oral hypoglycemic agent and insulin) to manage the blood glucose levels of people with Type 2 diabetes.

complications

Harmful effects of diabetes such as damage to the eyes, heart, blood vessels, nervous system, teeth and gums, feet and skin, or kidneys. Studies show that keeping blood glucose, blood pressure, and low-density lipoprotein cholesterol levels close to normal can help prevent or delay these problems.

conventional therapy

A term used in clinical trials where one group receives treatment for diabetes in which A1c and blood glucose levels are kept at levels based on current practice guidelines. However, the goal is not to keep blood glucose levels as close to normal as possible, as is done in intensive therapy. Conventional therapy includes use of medication, meal planning, and exercise, along with regular visits to health care providers.

coronary heart disease

Heart disease caused by narrowing of the arteries that supply blood to the heart. If the blood supply is cut off, the result is a heart attack.

Co-trimoxazole

A combination of trimethoprim and sulfamethoxazole, a sulfa drug. It can kill bacteria that cause various infections, including infections of the urinary tract, lungs (pneumonia), ears, and intestines. It also is used to treat "travelers" diarrhea. Antibiotics will not work for colds, flu, or other viral infections. Also know as Bactrim and/or Septra.

creatinine

A waste product from protein in the diet and from the muscles of the body. Creatinine is removed from the body by the kidneys; as kidney disease progresses, the level of creatinine in the blood increases.

D

Daclizumab

A drug that belongs to a group of medicines known as immunosuppressive agents. It is used to lower the body's natural immunity in patients who receive transplants. When a patient receives a transplant, the body's white blood cells will try to get rid of (reject) the transplanted cells. Daclizumab works by preventing the white blood cells from getting rid of the transplanted cells. The effect of Daclizumab on the white blood cells may also reduce the body's ability to fight infections. Also known as Zenapax.

dawn phenomenon

The early morning (4 a.m. to 8 a.m.) rise in blood glucose level.

dehydration

The loss of too much body fluid. This can occur through frequent urinating, sweating, diarrhea, or vomiting.

dermatology

A branch of science dealing with the skin, its structure, functions, and diseases.

dermatologist

A physician specializing in diseases of the skin.

dextrose, also called glucose

Simple sugar found in blood that serves as the body's main source of energy.

Diabetes Control and Complications Trial (DCCT)

A study by the National Institute of Diabetes and Digestive and Kidney Diseases, conducted from 1983 to 1993 in people with Type 1 diabetes. The study showed that intensive therapy compared to conventional therapy significantly helped prevent or delay diabetes complications. Intensive therapy included multiple daily insulin injections or the use of an insulin pump with multiple blood glucose readings each day. Complications followed in the study included diabetic retinopathy, neuropathy, and nephropathy, and all three were reduced by intensive therapy.

diabetes educator

A health care professional who teaches people who have diabetes how to manage their diabetes. Some diabetes educators are certified diabetes educators (CDES). Diabetes educators are found in hospitals, physician offices, managed care organizations, home health care, and other settings.

diabetes insipidus

A condition characterized by frequent and heavy urination, excessive thirst, and an overall feeling of weakness. This condition may be caused by a defect in the pituitary gland or in the kidney. In diabetes insipidus, blood glucose levels are normal.

diabetes mellitus

A condition characterized by hyperglycemia resulting from the body's inability to use blood glucose for energy. In Type 1 diabetes, the pancreas no longer makes insulin and therefore blood glucose cannot enter the cells to be used for energy. In Type 2 diabetes, either the pancreas does not make enough insulin or the body is unable to use insulin correctly.

Diabetes Prevention Program (DPP)

A study by the National Institute of Diabetes and Digestive and Kidney Diseases conducted from 1998 to 2001 in people at high risk for Type 2 diabetes. All study participants had impaired glucose tolerance, also called pre-diabetes, and were overweight. The study showed that people who lost 5 to 7 percent of their body weight through a low-fat, low-calorie diet and moderate exercise (usually walking for 30 minutes 5 days a week) reduced their risk of getting Type 2 diabetes by 58 percent. Participants who received treatment with the oral diabetes drug metformin reduced their risk of getting Type 2 diabetes by 31 percent.

diabetic diarrhea

Loose stools, fecal incontinence, or both that result from an overgrowth of bacteria in the small intestine and diabetic neuropathy in the intestines. This nerve damage can also result in constipation.

diabetic ketoacidosis (DKA)

An emergency condition in which extremely high blood glucose levels, along with a severe lack of insulin, result in the breakdown of body fat for energy and an accumulation of ketone acids in the blood and urine. Signs of DKA are nausea and vomiting, stomach pain, fruity breath odor, and rapid breathing. Untreated DKA can lead to coma and death.

diabetic retinopathy

Diabetic eye disease; damage to the small blood vessels in the retina. Loss of vision may result.

diabetologist

A doctor who specializes in treating people with diabetes.

diagnosis

The determination of a disease from its signs and symptoms.

dilated eye exam

A test done by an eye care specialist in which the pupil (the black center) of the eye is temporarily enlarged with eye drops to allow the specialist to see the inside of the eye more easily.

dietitian

A health care professional who advises people about meal planning, weight control and diabetes management. A registered dietitian (RD) has more training.

E

edema

Swelling caused by excess fluid in the body.

electrocardiograph (ekg)

An instrument for recording the changes of electrical potential occurring during the heartbeat used especially in diagnosing abnormalities of heat action.

endocrine gland

A group of specialized cells that release hormones into the blood. For example, the islets in the pancreas, which secrete insulin, are endocrine glands.

endocrinologist

A doctor who treats people who have endocrine gland problems such as diabetes.

enzyme

Protein made by the body that brings about a chemical reaction, for example, the enzymes produced by the gut to aid digestion.

euglycemia

A normal level of glucose in the blood.

exchange lists

One of several approaches for diabetes meal planning. Foods are categorized into three groups based on their nutritional content. Lists provide the serving sizes for carbohydrates, meat and meat alternatives, and fats. These lists allow for substitution for different groups to keep the nutritional content fixed.

F

fasting blood glucose test

A check of a person's blood glucose level after the person has not eaten for 8 to 12 hours (usually overnight). This test is used to diagnose pre-diabetes and diabetes. It is also used to monitor people with diabetes.

fat

1. One of the three main nutrients in food. Foods that provide fat are butter, margarine, salad dressing, oil, nuts, meat, poultry, fish and some dairy products. 2. Excess calories are stored as body fat, providing the body with a reserve supply of energy and other functions.

flexible sigmoidoscopy

A technique that enables the physician to look at the inside of the large intestine from the rectum through the last part of the colon, called the sigmoid or descending colon. Used to look for early signs of cancer in the descending colon and rectum.

fructose

A sugar that occurs naturally in fruits and honey.

G

gangrene

The death of body tissue, most often caused by a lack of blood flow and infection. It can lead to amputation.

gastroparesis

A form of neuropathy that affects the stomach. Digestion of food may be incomplete or delayed, resulting in nausea, vomiting, or bloating, making blood glucose control difficult.

geneticist

A specialist or expert in genetics.

genetics

A branch of biology that deals with the heredity and variation of organisms.

gestational diabetes mellitus (GDM)

A type of diabetes mellitus that develops only during pregnancy and usually disappears upon delivery, but increases the risk that the mother will develop diabetes later. GDM is managed with meal planning, activity, and in some cases, insulin.

gland

A group of cells that secrete substances. Endocrine glands secrete hormones. Exocrine glands secrete salt, enzymes, and water.

glargine insulin

A type of very long-acting insulin that works slowly over about 24 hours. On average, Lantus insulin starts to lower blood glucose levels within 1 hour after injection and keeps working evenly for 24 hours.

glaucoma

An increase in fluid pressure inside the eye that, if not treated, may lead to loss of vision.

glucagon

A hormone produced by the alpha cells in the pancreas. It raises blood glucose. An injectable form of glucagon, available by prescription, may be used to treat severe hypoglycemia.

glucose

One of the simplest forms of sugar.

glucose tablets

Chewable tablets made of pure glucose used for treating hypoglycemia.

glycemic index

A ranking of carbohydrate-containing foods, based on the food's effect on blood glucose compared with a standard reference food.

glycogen

The form of glucose found in the liver and muscles.

glycosuria

The presence of glucose in the urine.

H

half-life

The time required for half of something to undergo a process. That is, the time required for half the amount of a medication or radioactive tracer to be eliminated by natural processes. For example, consider a drug with a half-life of 1 day: One day after taking the drug, half of it remains and half is eliminated from the body. After the second day, half of the remainder is eliminated leaving one-quarter of the original amount. And so on.

HMO

A health maintenance organization provides comprehensive health care to voluntarily enrolled individuals and families in a particular geographic area by member physicians with limited referral to outside specialists, and that is financed by fixed periodic payments determined in advance and by co-payments for most services.

HDL cholesterol (high-density-lipoprotein cholesterol)

A fat found in the blood that takes extra cholesterol from the tissues, via the blood to the liver for removal. Sometimes called "good" cholesterol.

Hemoglobin A1c

See "A1c".

heredity

The passing of a trait from parent to child.

honeymoon phase

Temporary remission of hyperglycemia that occurs in some people newly diagnosed with Type 1 diabetes, when insulin secreted from their pancreas is sufficient to control the blood sugar. The honeymoon usually lasts a few months, or less.

hormone

A chemical produced in one part of the body and released into the blood to trigger or regulate particular functions of the body. For example, insulin is a hormone made in the pancreas that tells other cells when to use glucose for energy. Synthetic hormones, made for use as medicines, can be the same or different from those made in the body.

human leukocyte antigens (HLA)

Proteins located on the surface of the cell that help the immune system identify the cell either as one belonging to the body or as one from outside the body. Some patterns of these proteins may mean increased risk of developing Type 1 diabetes.

hyperglycemia

Excessive blood glucose. Fasting hyperglycemia is blood glucose above a desirable level after a person has fasted for at least 8 hours. Postprandial hyperglycemia is blood glucose above a desirable level 1 to 2 hours after a person has eaten.

hypertension

A condition present when blood flows through the blood vessels with a force greater than normal. Also called high blood pressure. Hypertension can strain the heart, damage blood vessels, and increase the risk of heart attack, stroke, kidney problems, and death.

hypoglycemia

A condition that occurs when one's blood glucose is lower than normal, usually less than 70 mg/dL. Signs include hunger, nervousness, shakiness, perspiration, dizziness or light-headedness, sleepiness, and confusion. If left untreated, hypoglycemia may lead to unconsciousness. Hypoglycemia is treated by consuming a carbohydrate-rich food such as a glucose tablet or juice. It may also be treated with an injection of glucagon if the person is unconscious or unable to swallow. Also called an insulin reaction.

hypoglycemia unawareness

A state in which a person does not feel or recognize the symptoms of hypoglycemia. People who have frequent episodes of hypoglycemia may no longer experience the typical warning signs.

Humalog

A rapid-acting human insulin. Humalog starts to work almost immediately, compared to regular insulin which requires about 30 minutes to begin to work. Humalog can be injected right before a meal, or even immediately *after* a meal.

I

IDDM (insulin-dependent diabetes mellitus)

Former term for Type 1 diabetes.

immune system

The body's system for protecting itself from viruses and bacteria or any "foreign" substances.

immunosuppressant

A drug that suppresses the natural immune responses. Immunosuppressants are given to transplant patients to prevent organ rejection or to patients with autoimmune diseases to limit the autoimmune attack.

impaired fasting glucose (IFG)

A condition in which a blood glucose test, taken after an 8- to 12-hour fast, shows a level of glucose higher than normal but not high enough for a diagnosis of diabetes. IFG, also called pre-diabetes, is a level of 110 mg/dL to 125 mg/dL. Most people with pre-diabetes are at increased risk for developing Type 2 diabetes.

impaired glucose tolerance (IGT)

A condition in which blood glucose levels are higher than normal but are not high enough for a diagnosis of diabetes. IGT, also called pre-diabetes, is a level of 140 mg/dL to 199 mg/dL 2 hours after the start of an oral glucose tolerance test. Most people with pre-diabetes are at increased risk for developing Type 2 diabetes. Other names for IGT that are no longer used are "borderline," "subclinical," "chemical," or "latent" diabetes.

implantable insulin pump

A small pump placed inside the body to deliver insulin in response to remote-control commands from the user.

incidence

A measure of how often a disease occurs; the number of new cases of a disease among a certain group of people for a certain period of time.

inhaled insulin

An experimental treatment for taking insulin using a portable device that allows a person to breathe in insulin.

injection

Inserting liquid medication or nutrients into the body with a syringe. A person with diabetes may use short needles or pinch the skin and inject at an angle to avoid an intramuscular injection of insulin.

injection site rotation

Changing the places on the body where insulin is injected. Rotation prevents the formation of fat deposits induced by insulin.

injection sites

Places on the body where insulin is usually injected.

insulin

A hormone that helps the body use glucose for energy. The beta cells of the pancreas make insulin. When the body cannot make enough insulin, it is taken by injection or through use of an insulin pump.

insulin adjustment

A change in the amount of insulin a person with diabetes takes based on factors such as meal planning, activity and blood glucose levels.

insulin pen

A device for injecting insulin that looks like a fountain pen and holds replaceable cartridges of insulin. Also available in disposable form.

insulin pump

An insulin-delivering device about the size of a deck of cards that can be worn on a belt or kept in a pocket. An insulin pump connects to narrow, flexible plastic tubing that ends with a needle inserted just under the skin. Users set the pump to give a steady trickle or basal amount of insulin continuously throughout the day. Pumps also can be triggered by the user to release bolus doses of insulin (several units at a time) at meals and at times when blood glucose is too high.

insulin reaction

Occurs when the level of glucose in the blood is too low (at or below 70 mg/dL). Also known as hypoglycemia.

insulin receptors

Areas on the outer part of a cell that allow the cell to bind with insulin in the blood. When the insulin receptor on the cell surface binds with insulin, the cell can take glucose from the blood and use it for energy.

insulin resistance

The body's inability to respond to and use the insulin it produces. Insulin resistance may be linked to obesity, hypertension, and high levels of fat in the blood.

insulin-dependent diabetes mellitus (IDDM)

Former term for Type 1 diabetes.

intensive therapy

A treatment for diabetes in which blood glucose is kept as close to normal as possible through frequent injections or use of an insulin pump, meal planning, adjustment of medicines, exercise based on blood glucose test results, and frequent contact with a person's health care team.

intermediate-acting insulin

A type of insulin that starts to lower blood glucose within 1 to 2 hours after injection and has its strongest effect 6 to 12 hours after injection, depending on the type used. See NPH insulin.

intramuscular injection

Inserting liquid medication into a muscle with a syringe. Glucagon may be given by subcutaneous or intramuscular injection for hypoglycemia.

intravenous

Situated within, performed within, occurring within, or administered by entering a vein; an intravenous solution.

islet cell autoantibodies (ICA)

Proteins found in the blood of people newly diagnosed with Type 1 diabetes. They are also found in people who may be developing Type 1 diabetes. The presence of ICA indicates that the body's immune system has been damaging beta cells in the pancreas.

islet transplantation

Moving the islets from a donor pancreas into a person whose pancreas has stopped producing insulin. Beta cells in the islets make the insulin that the body needs for using blood glucose.

islets

Groups of cells located in the pancreas that make hormones that help the body break down and use food. For example, alpha cells make glucagon and beta cells make insulin. Also called islets of Langerhans.

J

juvenile diabetes

Former term for insulin-dependent diabetes mellitus (IDDM), or Type 1 diabetes.

K

ketone

A chemical produced when there is a shortage of insulin in the blood and the body breaks down body fat for energy. High levels of ketones can lead to diabetic ketoacidosis and coma. Sometimes referred to as ketone bodies.

ketosis

A ketone buildup in the body that may lead to diabetic ketoacidosis. Signs of ketosis are nausea, vomiting, and stomach pain.

kidney failure

A chronic condition in which the body retains fluid and harmful wastes build up because the kidneys no longer work properly. A person with kidney failure needs dialysis or a kidney transplant. Also called end-stage renal disease or ESRD.

kidneys

The two bean-shaped organs that filter wastes from the blood and form urine. The kidneys are located near the middle of the back. They send urine to the bladder.

L

lancet

A spring-loaded device used to prick the skin with a small needle to obtain a drop of blood for blood glucose monitoring.

Lantus insulin

A type of very long-acting insulin that works slowly over about 24 hours. On average, Lantus insulin starts to lower blood glucose levels within 1 hour after injection and keeps working evenly for 24 hours.

laser surgery treatment

A type of therapy that uses a strong beam of light to treat a damaged area. The beam of light is called a laser. A laser is sometimes used to seal blood vessels in the eye of a person with diabetes. See photocoagulation.

latent autoimmune diabetes in adults (LADA)

A condition in which Type 1 diabetes develops in adults.

lente insulin

A rapid-acting insulin that starts to lower blood glucose within 5 to 10 minutes after injection and has its strongest effect 30 minutes to 3 hours after injection.

Lovenox

A low molecular heparin.

LDL cholesterol (low-density lipoprotein cholesterol)

A fat found in the blood that takes cholesterol around the body to where it is needed for cell repair and also deposits it on the inside of artery walls. Sometimes called "bad" cholesterol.

lipid

A term for fat in the body. Lipids can be broken down by the body and used for energy.

lipid profile

A blood test that measures total cholesterol, triglycerides, and HDL cholesterol. LDL cholesterol is then calculated from the results. A lipid profile is one measure of a person's risk of cardiovascular disease.

Lisinopril

A drug used to treat high blood pressure and heart failure. It decreases certain chemicals that tighten the blood vessels, so blood flows more smoothly and the heart can pump blood more efficiently. Also known as Zestril.

lispro insulin

A rapid-acting insulin that starts to lower blood glucose within 5 to 10 minutes after injection and has its strongest effect 30 minutes to 3 hours after injection.

liver

An organ in the body that changes food into energy, removes alcohol and poisons from the blood, and makes bile, a substance that breaks down fats and helps rid the body of wastes.

long-acting insulin

A type of insulin that starts to lower blood glucose within 4 to 6 hours after injection and has its strongest effect in 10 to 18 hours. It keeps working for 24 to 28 hours after injection. See ultralente insulin.

M

macrosomia

Abnormally large; in diabetes, refers to abnormally large babies that may be born to women with diabetes.

macrovascular disease

Disease of the large blood vessels, such as those found in the heart. Lipids and blood clots build up in the large blood vessels and can cause atherosclerosis, coronary heart disease, stroke, and peripheral vascular disease.

metabolic syndrome

The tendency of several conditions to occur together, including obesity, insulin resistance, diabetes or pre-diabetes, hypertension, and high lipids.

metabolism

The term for the way cells change food chemically so that it can be used to store or use energy and make the proteins, fats, and sugars needed by the body.

metformin

An oral medicine used to treat Type 2 diabetes. It lowers blood glucose by reducing the amount of glucose produced by the liver and helping the body respond better to the insulin made in the pancreas. Belongs to the class of medicines called biguanides. Brand names: Glucophage, Glucophage XR; an ingredient in Glucovance.

Mg/dL

Milligrams per deciliter, a unit of measure that shows the concentration of a substance in a specific amount of fluid. In the United States, blood glucose test results are reported as mg/dL. Medical journals and other countries use millimoles per liter (mmol/l). To convert to mg/dL from mmol/l, multiply mmol/l by 18. Example: 10 mmol/l x18 = 180 mg/dL.

microaneurysm

A small swelling that forms on the side of tiny blood vessels. These small swellings may break and allow blood to leak into nearby tissue. People with diabetes may get microaneurysms in the retina of the eye.

microvascular disease

Disease of the smallest blood vessels, such as those found in the eyes, nerves, and kidneys. The walls of the vessels become abnormally thick but weak. Then they bleed, leak protein, and slow the flow of blood to the cells.

mixed dose

A combination of two types of insulin in one injection. Usually a rapid- or short-acting insulin is combined with a longer acting insulin (such as NPH insulin) to provide both short-term and long-term control of blood glucose levels.

N

NICU

Neonatal intensive care unit

nephropathy

Disease of the kidneys. Hyperglycemia and hypertension can damage the kidneys' glomeruli. When the kidneys are damaged, protein leaks out of the kidneys into the urine. Damaged kidneys can no longer remove waste and extra fluids from the bloodstream.

neuropathy

Disease of the nervous system. The three major forms in people with diabetes are peripheral neuropathy, autonomic neuropathy, and mononeuropathy. The most common form is peripheral neuropathy, which affects mainly the legs and feet.

noninsulin-dependent diabetes mellitus (NIDDM)

Former term for Type 2 diabetes.

noninvasive blood glucose monitoring

Measuring blood glucose without pricking the finger to obtain a blood sample.

NPH insulin

A type of intermediate-acting insulin; NPH stands for neutral protamine hagedorn. On average, NPH insulin starts to lower blood glucose within 1 to 2 hours after injection. It has its strongest effect 6 to 12 hours after injection. Also called N insulin.

nutritionist

A person with training in nutrition.

O

obesity

A condition in which a greater than normal amount of fat is in the body; more severe than overweight; having a body mass index of 30 kg/m2 or more.

obstetrician

A doctor who treats pregnant women and delivers babies.

ophthalmologist

A medical doctor who diagnoses and treats eye diseases and eye disorders. Ophthalmologists can also prescribe glasses and contact lenses.

optician

A health care professional who dispenses glasses and lenses. An optician also makes and fits contact lenses.

optometrist

A primary eye care provider who prescribes glasses and contact lenses. Optometrists can diagnose and treat certain eye conditions and diseases.

oral glucose tolerance test (OGTT)

A test to diagnose diabetes. The oral glucose tolerance test is given by a health care professional after an overnight fast. A blood sample is taken, then the patient drinks a high-glucose beverage. Blood samples are taken at intervals for 2 to 3 hours. Test results are compared with a standard and show how the body uses glucose over time.

oral hypoglycemic agents

Medicines taken by mouth by people with Type 2 diabetes to keep blood glucose levels as close to normal as possible. Classes of oral hypoglycemic agents are alpha-glucosidase inhibitors, biguanides, d-phenylalanine derivatives, meglitinides, sulfonylureas, and thiazolidinediones.

overweight

An above-normal body weight; having a body mass index of 25 to 29.9 kg/m2.

P

pancreas

An organ that makes insulin and enzymes for digestion. The pancreas is located behind the lower part of the stomach and is about the size of a hand.

pancreas transplantation

A surgical procedure to take a healthy whole or partial pancreas from a donor and place it into a person with diabetes.

pediatric endocrinologist

A doctor who treats children who have endocrine gland problems such as diabetes.

peripheral neuropathy

Nerve damage that affects the feet, legs, or hands. Peripheral neuropathy causes pain, numbness, or a tingling feeling.

peripheral vascular disease (PVD)

A disease of the large blood vessels of the arms, legs, and feet. PVD may occur when major blood vessels in these areas are blocked and do not receive enough blood. The signs of PVD are aching pains and slow-healing foot sores.

pharmacist

A health care professional who prepares and distributes medicine to people. Pharmacists also give information on medicines.

photocoagulation

A treatment for diabetic retinopathy. A strong beam of light (laser) is used to seal off bleeding blood vessels in the eye and to burn away extra blood vessels that should not have grown there.

pioglitazone

An oral medicine used to treat Type 2 diabetes. It helps insulin take glucose from the blood into the cells for energy by making cells more sensitive to insulin. Belongs to the class of medicines called thiazolidinediones. (Brand name: Actos.)

polydipsia

Excessive thirst; may be a sign of diabetes.

polyphagia

Excessive hunger; may be a sign of diabetes.

polyuria

Excessive urination; may be a sign of diabetes.

postprandial blood glucose

The blood glucose level taken 1 to 2 hours after eating.

pre-diabetes

Former name for a condition in which blood glucose levels are higher than normal but are not high enough for a diagnosis of diabetes. People with pre-diabetes are at increased risk for developing Type 2 diabetes and for heart disease and stroke. Now referred to as impaired glucose tolerance and/or impaired fasting glucose.

premixed insulin

A commercially produced combination of two different types of insulin.

preprandial blood glucose

The blood glucose level taken before eating.

prevalence

The number of people in a given group or population who are reported to have a disease.

proinsulin

The substance made first in the pancreas and then broken into several pieces to become insulin.

proliferative retinopathy

A condition in which fragile new blood vessels grow along the retina and in the vitreous humor of the eye.

protein

1. One of the three main nutrients in food. Foods that provide protein include meat, poultry, fish, cheese, milk, dairy products, eggs, and dried beans. 2. Proteins also are used in the body for cell structure, hormones such as insulin, and other functions.

proteinuria

The presence of protein in the urine, indicating that the kidneys are not working properly.

R

radiologist

A physician specializing in the use of radiant energy for diagnostic and therapeutic purposes.

rapid-acting insulin

A type of insulin that starts to lower blood glucose within 5 to 10 minutes after injection and has its strongest effect 30 minutes to 3 hours after injection. Types of rapid-acting insulin include Lispro and lennte insulin and Humalog.

rebound hyperglycemia

A swing to a high level of glucose in the blood after a low level. See Somogyi effect.

regular insulin

A type of short-acting insulin. On average, regular insulin starts to lower blood glucose within 30 minutes after injection. It has its strongest effect 2 to 5 hours after injection but keeps working for 5 to 8 hours after injection. Also called R insulin.

renal

Having to do with the kidneys. A renal disease is a disease of the kidneys. Renal failure means the kidneys have stopped working.

renal threshold of glucose

The blood glucose concentration at which the kidneys start to excrete glucose into the urine.

retina

The light-sensitive layer of tissue that lines the back of the eye.

retinopathy

Diabetic eye disease; damage to the small blood vessels in the retina. Loss of vision may result.

risk factor

Anything that raises the chances of a person developing a disease.

S

seizure

Characterized by loss of consciousness, falling down, loss of bowel or bladder control, and rhythmic convulsions.

self-management

In diabetes, the ongoing process of managing diabetes. Includes meal planning, planned physical activity, blood glucose monitoring, taking diabetes medicines, handling episodes of illness and of low and high blood glucose, managing diabetes when traveling, and more. The person with diabetes designs his or her own self-management treatment plan in consultation with a variety of health care professionals such as doctors, nurses, dietitians, pharmacists, and others.

short-acting insulin

A type of insulin that starts to lower blood glucose within 30 minutes after injection and has its strongest effect 2 to 5 hours after injection but keeps working 5 to 8 hours after injection. See regular insulin.

side effects

The unintended action(s) of a drug.

Simvastatin

A drug used with diet changes (restriction of cholesterol and fat intake) to reduce the amount of cholesterol and certain fatty substances in your blood. Also know as Zocor.

Sirolimus

A drug in a class of medications called immunosuppressants. It works by suppressing the body's immune system. Also know as rapamune.

sliding scale

A set of instructions for adjusting insulin on the basis of blood glucose test results, meals, or activity levels.

Somogyi effect, also called rebound hyperglycemia

When the blood glucose level swings high following hypoglycemia. The Somogyi effect may follow an untreated hypoglycemic episode during the night and is caused by the release of stress hormones.

split mixed dose

Division of a prescribed daily dose of insulin into two or more injections combining a short acting and a longer acting insulin given over the course of the day.

starch

Another name for carbohydrate, one of the three main nutrients in food.

statins

A class of medications that work by preventing the production of cholesterol in the body.

stroke

Condition caused by damage to blood vessels in the brain; may cause loss of ability to speak or to move parts of the body.

subcutaneous injection

Putting a fluid into the tissue under the skin with a needle and syringe.

sugar

1. A class of carbohydrates with a sweet taste, including glucose, fructose and sucrose. 2. A term used to refer to blood glucose.

sugar diabetes

Former term for diabetes mellitus.

syringe

A device used to inject medications or other liquids into body tissues. The syringe for insulin has a hollow plastic tube with a plunger inside and a needle on the end.

T

tacrolimus

A drug in a class of medications called immunosuppressants used to prevent rejection of transplants. Also called Prograf and FK506.

team management

A diabetes treatment approach in which medical care is provided by a team of health care professionals including a doctor, a dietitian, a nurse, a diabetes educator, and others. The team advises the person with diabetes.

thallium stress test

A nuclear scanning test or myocardial perfusion imaging test. It shows how well blood flows to the heart muscle. It is usually done along with an exercise stress test on a treadmill. When the patient reaches his or her maximum level of exercise, a small amount of a radioactive substance called thallium is injected into the bloodstream. Then the patient lies down on a special table under a camera ("gamma camera") that can see the thallium and make pictures. The thallium mixes with the blood in the bloodstream and in the heart's arteries and enters heart muscle cells. If a part of the heart muscle doesn't receive a normal blood supply, less than a normal amount of thallium will be in those heart muscle cells. The first pictures are made shortly after the exercise test and show blood flow to the heart during exercise. The heart is "stressed" during the exercise test—thus the name "stress test." The patient then lies quietly for 2-3 hours and another series of pictures is made. These show blood flow to the heart muscle during rest.

triglyceride

The storage form of fat in the body. High triglyceride levels may occur when diabetes is out of control.

Type 1 diabetes

A condition characterized by high blood glucose levels caused by a total or near-total lack of insulin. Occurs when the body's immune system attacks the insulin-producing beta cells in the pancreas and destroys them. The pancreas then produces little or no insulin. Type 1 diabetes develops most often in young people but can appear in adults.

Type 2 diabetes

A condition characterized by high blood glucose levels caused by either a relative lack of insulin or the body's inability to use insulin efficiently. Type 2 diabetes develops most often in middle-aged and older adults but can appear in young people.

U

ulcer

A deep open sore or break in the skin.

ultralente insulin

A type of long-acting insulin. On average, ultralente insulin starts to lower blood glucose within 4 to 6 hours after injection. It has its strongest effect in 10 to 18 hours, but keeps working for 24 to 28 hours after injection. Also called U insulin.

unit of insulin

The basic measure of insulin. U-100 insulin means 100 units of insulin per milliliter (ml) or cubic centimeter (cc) of solution. Most insulin made today in the United States is U-100.

United Kingdom Prospective Diabetes Study (UKPDS)

A study in England, conducted from 1977 to 1997 in people with Type 2 diabetes. The study showed that if people lowered their blood glucose, they lowered their risk of eye disease and kidney damage. In addition, those with Type

2 diabetes and hypertension who lowered their blood pressure also reduced their risk of stroke, eye damage, and death from long-term complications.

urea

A waste product found in the blood that results from the normal breakdown of protein in the liver. Urea is normally removed from the blood by the kidneys and then excreted in the urine.

uremia

The illness associated with the buildup of urea in the blood because the kidneys do not work effectively. Symptoms include nausea, vomiting, loss of appetite, weakness, and mental confusion.

urine

The liquid waste product filtered from the blood by the kidneys, stored in the bladder, and expelled from the body by the act of urinating.

urine testing

Also called urinalysis; a test of a urine sample to diagnose diseases of the urinary system and other body systems. Urine may also be checked for signs of bleeding. Some tests use a single urine sample. For others, 24-hour collection may be needed. And sometimes a sample is "cultured" to see exactly what type of bacteria grows.

V

vascular

Relating to the body's blood vessels.

viscera

A collective term used to describe the internal organs.

vein

A blood vessel that carries blood to the heart.

very-long-acting insulin

A type of insulin that starts to lower blood glucose within 1 hour after injection and keeps working evenly for 24 hours. See glargine and Lantus insulin.

W

wound care

Steps taken to ensure that a wound such as a foot ulcer heals correctly. People with diabetes need to take special precautions so wounds do not become infected.

INTERNET RESOURCES

ADA

American Diabetes Association (www.diabetes.org)

JDRF

Juvenile Diabetes Research Association (www.jdrf.org)

NIH

National Institutes of Health (www.nih.gov)

NIDDK

National Institute of Digestive, Diabetes and Kidney Diseases (www.nih/niddk.gov)

Diabetes Station (www.diabetesstation.com)

Diabetes Portal (www.diabetesportal.com)

Diabetes Wellness Network (www.diabeteswellness.org)

Immune Tolerance Network (www.immunetolerance.org)

Clinical Trials (www.clinicaltrails.gov)

NDIC

National Diabetes Information Clearinghouse (http://diabetes.niddk.nih.gov/about/index.htm)

Email: ndic@info.niddk.nih.gov

1 Information Way

Bethesda, MD 20892-3560

The NDIC is a service of the NIDDK. The NIDDK is part of the National Institutes of Health under the U.S. Department of Health and Human Services. Established in 1978, the clearinghouse provides information about diabetes to people with diabetes and to their families, health care professionals, and the public. NDIC answers inquiries, develops and distributes publications, and works closely with professional and patient organizations and Government agencies to coordinate resources about diabetes.

ABOUT THE AUTHOR

Ellen Berty was troubled by diabetes complications of blackouts and seizures. Normally optimistic, she felt powerless as her illness got worse. Then she heard about an experimental procedure that offered great potential. She enrolled in a clinical trial and received an islet transplant at the National Institutes of Health. She tells the story of her extraordinary 40 year journey with Type 1 diabetes and her eventual cure. She instills hope that great progress is being made toward the ultimate goal of a universal cure for all who have diabetes.

www.ingramcontent.com/pod-product-compliance
Lightning Source LLC
Chambersburg PA
CBHW020430290526
45785CB00002B/779